Color Atlas of Differential Diagnosis of Hair Loss

Color Atlas of Differential Diagnosis of Hair Loss

David A. Whiting, M.D., F.A.C.P., F.R.C.P.(Ed.)
and
F. Lester Howsden, M.D.

David A. Whiting: Clinical Professor of Dermatology and Pediatrics,
University of Texas Southwestern Medical Center,
Dallas, Texas
Medical Director, Baylor Hair Research and
Treatment Center, Dallas, Texas

F. Lester Howsden: Clinical Associate Professor of Dermatology,
University of Texas Southwestern Medical Center,
Dallas, Texas

The Color Atlas of
Differential Diagnosis of Hair Loss

Canfield Publishing
218 Little Falls Road
Cedar Grove, NJ 07009

ISBN 0-9647749-0-9

Library of Congress Catalogue
Card Number: 95-70533

Table of Contents

Acknowledgements

We wish to express our thanks to Doris McGowan for her word processing skills in providing and editing various drafts of this manuscript and to Samuel E. Steinmetz, M.D. for proofing certain drafts.

We would also like to thank individuals who allowed use of their various photographs and graphics. These include Doctors K. P. Baker, F. P. Jordaan, M. Kerr, A. Lucky, V. H. Price, R. Savin, and E. J. Schulz.

We much appreciate the enthusiasm and expertise of Douglas Canfield, who has made this publication possible. Nancy Woodard of Canfield Scientific has been most helpful in coordinating our efforts.

Dedication

This book is dedicated to our wives, Harriet Whiting and Susan Howsden, without whose love and support the small accomplishments of our lives would have little meaning.

Preface

This color atlas represents an effort to provide a relatively concise presentation of the recognized patterns of alopecia. The extensive use of photographs of clinical examples, as well as photomicrographs of the associated histopathological findings, is intended to provide clarity and interest. Specifically, the use of horizontal sectioning of scalp biopsies and the resulting histopathologic findings are briefly described. We believe these histopathological findings for a number of the patterns of alopecia are described here for the first time in a single reference.

This atlas is intended for the use of dermatologists, particularly those who find the evaluation and treatment of hair loss to be somewhat tedious and often confusing. These individuals should find the chapter on "Assessment of Patient with Hair Loss" (Chapter 2) particularly helpful with its sample patient questionnaires, as well as descriptions of examination techniques.

We believe that family practitioners, internists, pediatricians, gynecologists, pathologists, physician assistants, as well as others, should find this a welcome reference to assist them in sorting out this sometimes complex subject. To make this atlas useful to such individuals we have endeavored to organize it in a logical fashion, to keep the text simple and concise, and to rely heavily on the use of color photographs.

Photographs and illustrations are identified by chapter and individual number. For example, the first figure in Chapter 1 is number 1.1. Photos in a series are further identified by a letter, indicating their position in the series, and by an arrow ➔ indicating succeeding photos, or by a square ■ indicating the end of a series. For example, 1.5a➔ is the first in a series and 1.5b■ is the end of that series. Please note that a photo series may begin on the left-facing page and continue on the right-facing page.

Introduction

I.1a

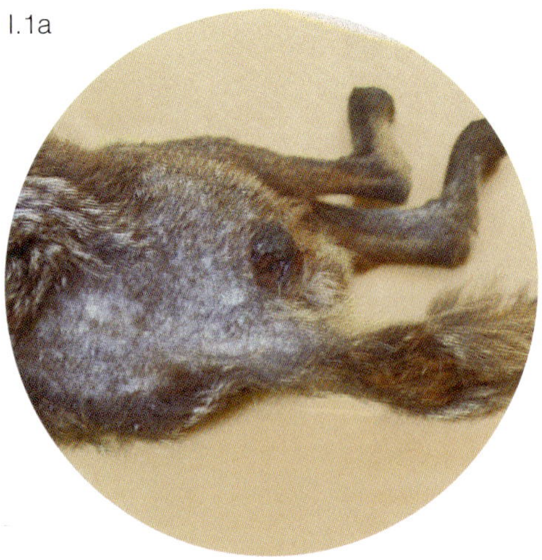

Intro.1

a. Patchy alopecia in a fox caused by scabetic mange. *(Courtesy of Kenneth P. Baker, DVD, Ph.D.)*

b. Red fox. *(Courtesy of Stephen M. Kerr, DVM)*

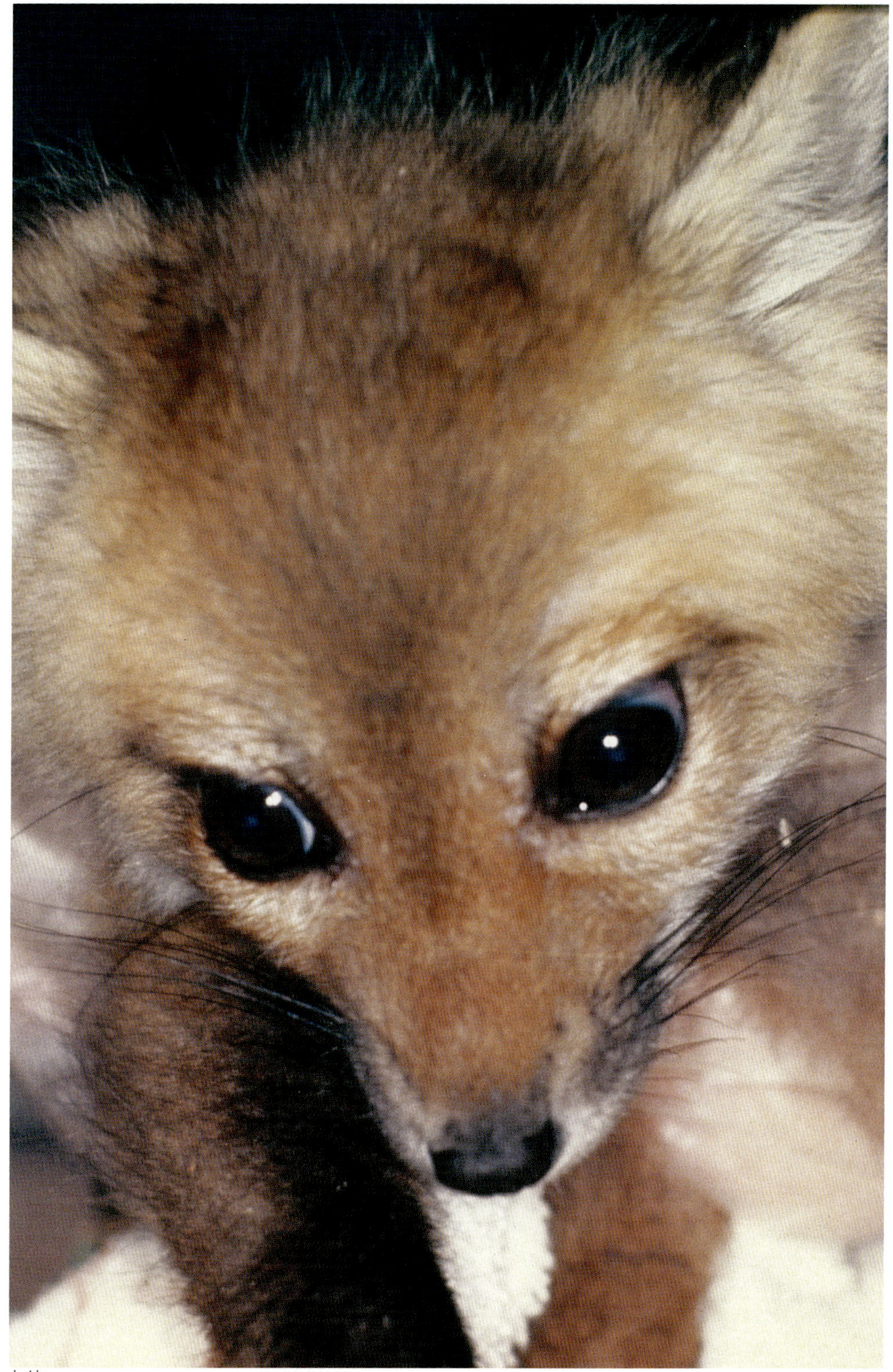

I.1b

Hair is one of the most variable characteristics of humans. It varies sufficiently in color, length, density, and shape to help define race. It provides an adornment or decoration, the development and maintenance of which supports entire industries.

The art of arranging hair into a pattern or design has been practiced from ancient times. Hair design has reflected social, religious, or economic status; however today, hair design revolves primarily around concepts of current fashion and particularly feminine beauty. With this most intricate relationship between hair and attractiveness it is easy to understand the urgency felt by patients with alopecia to have their hair restored.

Scalp hair provides protection from cold and mechanical injury, and is an effective natural sun screen for the scalp.

References to hair can be found in literature and religious writings throughout history. Samson lost his strength along with his locks (Judges 16:19). Absalom was left hanging in a great oak by his hair (2 Samuel 18:19). Rapunzel let down her shining locks of 20 ells' length (30 yards), and formed a ladder for the Witch to climb to the tower each night.

The absence of hair, alopecia, is of greatly variable cause and concern. The word alopecia is derived from the Greek word alopekia, meaning a fox. It refers to the patchy hair loss caused by scabetic mange (Figure Intro. 1a) which occurs in red foxes (Figure Intro. 1b). As used today alopecia refers to hair loss from any cause.

Significant alopecia poses cosmetic disturbance at the very least to the sufferer. The possibility of deferring loss or causing regrowth by chemical means has made it clear just how desperate many men and women are, both young and old, to retain or regain their natural scalp hair.

The correct diagnosis and treatment of the many forms of alopecia, which often have significance beyond cosmetic concerns, frequently confront the clinician. A better understanding of the causes and progression of alopecia is helpful for physician and patient alike. This atlas is designed to provide a concise description of recognized patterns of alopecia, as well as photographic examples of both clinical and histopathological findings in many cases. ■

Suggested Reading

Ackerman, A.B., deViragh, P.A., Chongchitnant, N.: *Neoplasms with Follicular Differentiation.* Philadelphia: Lea and Febiger, 1993.

Baccaredda–Boy, A., Monetti, G., Frey, J.R.: *Biopathology of Pattern Alopecia.* Basel: S. Karger, 1968.

Baden, H.P.: *Diseases of the Hair and Nails.* Chicago: Year Book, 1987.

Baran, R., Dawber, R.P.R., Levine, G.M.: *Color Atlas of the Hair, Scalp, and Nails.* St. Louis: Mosby–Year Book, 1992.

Bergsma, D., (Ed.): *Birth Defects, Original Article Series.* Baltimore: Williams and Wilkins, The National Foundation – March of Dimes (Skin, Hair and Nails, part XII), 1972.

Brown, A.C., (Ed.): *The First Human Hair Symposium.* New York: Medcom Press, 1974.

Brown, A.C., Crounse, R.G., (Eds.): *Hair, Trace Elements and Human Illness.* New York: Praeger, 1980.

Ferriman, D.: *Human Hair Growth in Health and Disease.* Springfield: Charles C. Thomas, 1971.

Jackson, G.T., McMurtry, C.W.: *Diseases of the Hair.* London, Henry Kimpton, 1913.

Kobori, T., Montagna, W., (Eds.): *Biology and Disease of the Hair.* Baltimore: University Park Press, 1976.

Mitchell, A.J., Krull, E.A., (Eds.): *Hair Disorders, Dermatology Clinics.* Philadelphia: W.B. Saunders, 1987:5(3).

Montagna, W., Dobson, R.L.: *Advances in Biology of Skin, Vol. IX: Hair Growth.* Oxford: Pergamon Press, 1969.

Montagna, W., Parakkal, P.F.: *The Structure and Function of the Skin (3rd ed.).* New York: Academic Press, 1974.

Norwood, O.T.: *Hair Transplant Surgery.* Springfield: Charles C. Thomas, 1973.

Olsen, E.A., (Ed.): *Disorders of Hair Growth. Diagnosis and Treatment.* New York: McGraw–Hill, 1994.

Orfanos, C.E., Happle, R., (Eds.): *Hair and Hair Diseases.* Berlin: Springer–Verlag, 1990.

Orfanos, C.E., Montagna, W., Stuttgen, G., (Eds.): *Hair Research: Status and Future Aspects.* Berlin: Springer–Verlag, 1981.

Rogers, G.E., Marshall, R.C., Rice, T.J., Ward, K.A., (Eds.): *The Biology of Wool and Hair.* London: Chapman and Hall, 1989.

Rook, A., Dawber, R.: *Diseases of the Hair and Scalp (2nd ed.).* Oxford: Blackwell Scientific Publications, 1991.

Van Neste, D., Lachapelle, J.M., Antoine, J.L.: *Trends in Human Hair Growth and Alopecia Research.* Dordrecht: Kluwer Academic Publishers, 1989.

Zviak, C., Ed.: *The Science of Hair Care.* New York: Marcel Dekker, Inc., 1986.

Normal Hair

The hair follicle consists of a permanent, upper segment composed of infundibulum and isthmus, and a transient, inferior segment composed of lower follicle and hair root (Figures 1.1, 1.2). The single hair fiber is a cellularly derived, tubular-shaped composite of keratin fibrils embedded in sulphur-rich material, enclosed in a protective cuticle. The follicular apparatus represents a miniature factory which almost continuously extrudes the end product, hair. Production is primarily determined by the hair matrix, a very rapidly dividing pool of cells surrounding the dermal papilla in the hair bulb (Figures 1.3, 1.4).

The rapidly dividing matrix cells differentiate into three different components of the developing hair. Centrally, the medullary cells arise at the apex of the dermal papilla and form granules and some randomly distributed filaments. Mature medullary cells may be seen in the central terminal hair; however, their complete absence in "vellus" and lanugo hair, as well as paucity in terminal hairs, raises doubts as to their significance. Cortical cells arise above and around the medullary cells and produce fibrillar proteins. As these cells mature more distally, the fibrillar proteins become densely packed into macrofibrils oriented to the long axis of the hair. The organized macrofibrils are in turn embedded in a structureless matrix which contains increasing sulphydryl groups as the upper keratogenous zone is reached. The nucleus of the cortical cell degenerates; however, a remnant of the cell mem-

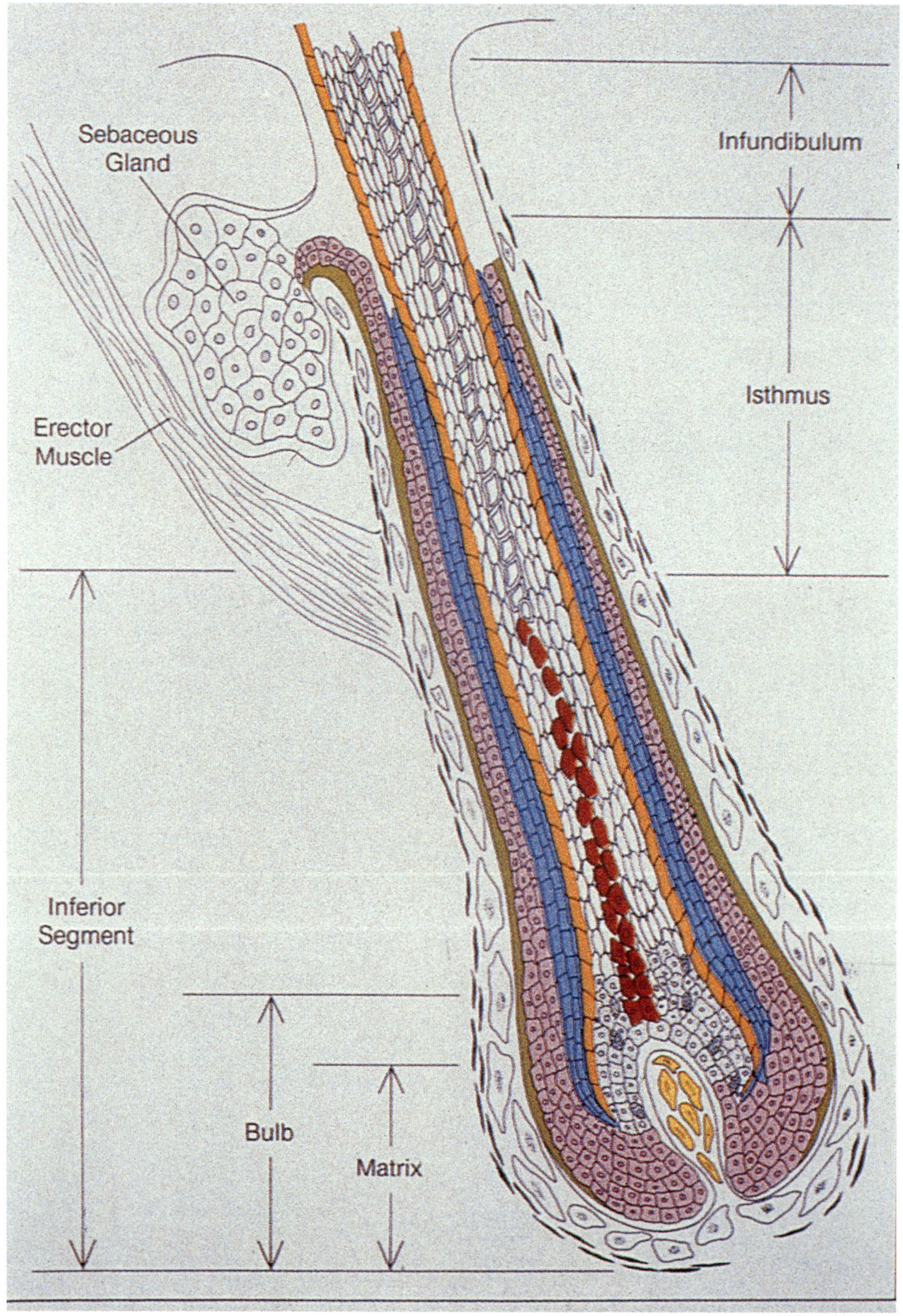

1.1

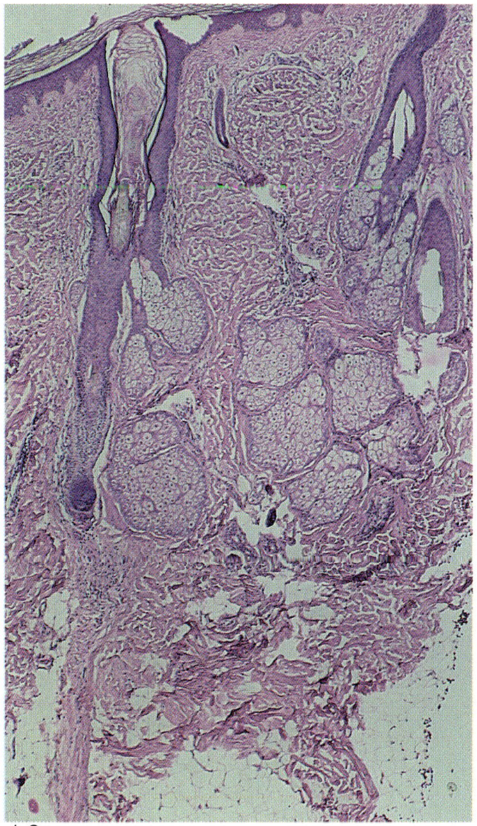

1.2

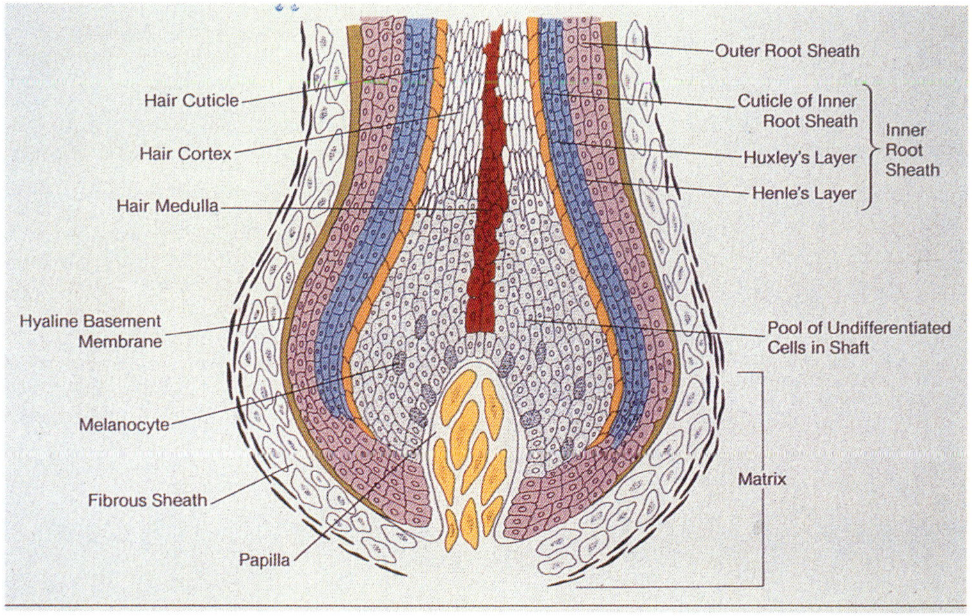

1.3

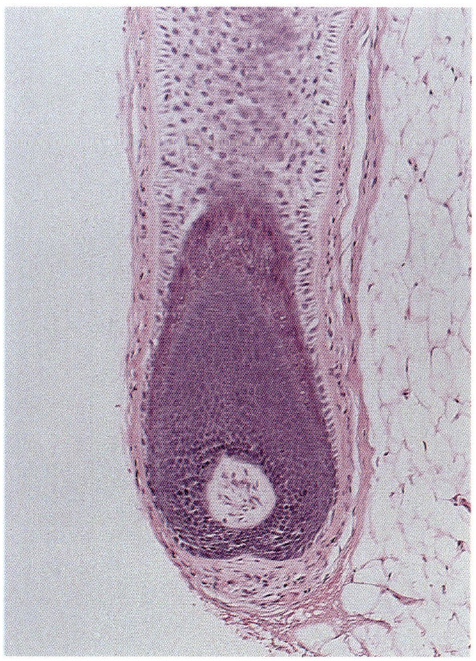

1.4

1.1
Diagram of normal hair follicle: The infundibulum, isthmus, and inferior segment are shown. *(Reprinted from Hospital Medicine, with permission.)*

1.2
Vertical section of biopsy of scalp skin: A hair follicle is shown with a streamer, or stela, visible below the hair bulb. Light microscopy (LM) x 40.

1.3
Diagram of normal anagen hair root: The dermal papilla is surrounded by hair bulb, and the cortex of the anagen hair shaft is enveloped by the hair cuticle, the cuticle of the inner root sheath, Huxley's layer, Henley's layer, outer root sheath, hyaline basement membrane, and fibrous sheath. *(Reprinted from Hospital Medicine, with permission.)*

1.4
Vertical section of hair root: The dermal papilla is surrounded by hair bulb matrix enveloped by outer root sheath, hyaline basement membrane, and fibrous sheath. LM x 100.

brane persists as the outline of the 'dead' cortical cells of the hair shaft. The cortex constitutes the major portion of hair and is responsible for its mechanical properties. Finally, cuticle cells develop outside the cortical cells and produce a non-fibrillar keratin. These cuticle cells flatten and form a six to 10 cell thick layer around the cortex. The most external cuticle cells overlap, with the free margins directed upwards toward the tip of the hair.

Other components of the follicular apparatus include the inner and outer root sheaths. While these play a role in molding the hair and allowing outward migration of the hair, they do not directly contribute structurally to the mature hair itself. However, cuticular cells of the inner root sheath are directed backwards to interlock with cuticular cells of the hair shaft, and prevent easy extraction of the hair. The inner root sheath is only present in the inferior segment of the hair follicle. It is formed in the hair bulb from the hair matrix and becomes fully keratinized in the lower follicle (Figures 1.5a,b). It disappears in the follicular isthmus, where it is replaced by trichilemmal keratin (Figure 1.6). The isthmus extends from the bulge area, which is the level of insertion of the arrector pili muscle, up to the level of entry of the sebaceous duct. The upper follicle or infundibulum extends from the sebaceous duct level to skin surface, and is lined by sur-

1.5
Vertical section of inferior segment of anagen hair follicle:

a. The hair shaft is enveloped by inner root sheath, outer root sheath, hyaline basement membrane, and fibrous sheath. Internal root sheath is fully keratinized in the upper portion of the inferior segment of the hair follicle. LM x 100.

b. The hair cortex on the left is enveloped by hair cuticle interdigitating with the keratinized cuticle of the inner root sheath, which in turn is enveloped by the keratinizing layer of Huxley, by the keratinized layer of Henley, and then outer root sheath, hyaline basement membrane and fibrous sheath. LM x 400.

1.6
Vertical section of inferior segment of anagen hair follicle and isthmus: The inner root sheath disappears at the level of the isthmus (←) and is replaced by trichilemmal keratin produced by the trichilemma or outer root sheath (→). LM x 100.

1.7
Vertical section of the infundibulum: The infundibulum is lined by epithelium continuous with the surface epidermis. LM x 100.

1.8
Vertical section of shortened inferior segment of catagen hair follicle: A catagen hair with a central column of trichilemmal cells shrinking by apoptosis is surrounded by a thickened hyaline basement membrane. LM x 400.

1.9
Vertical section of shortened inferior segment of telogen hair follicle: A club shaped telogen hair root is surrounded by trichilemmal keratin and retracted trichilemma. LM x 400.

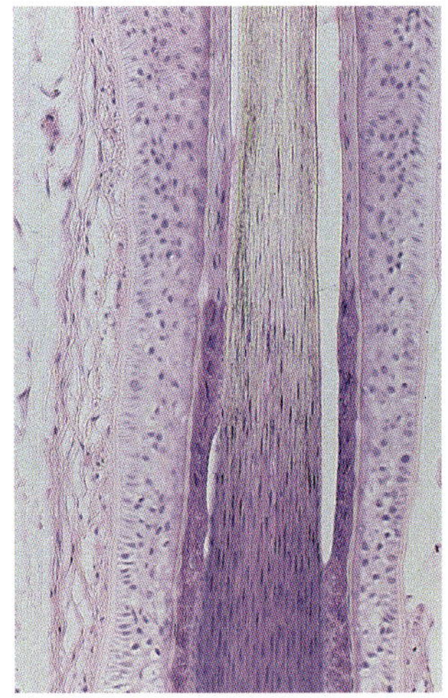

1.5a →

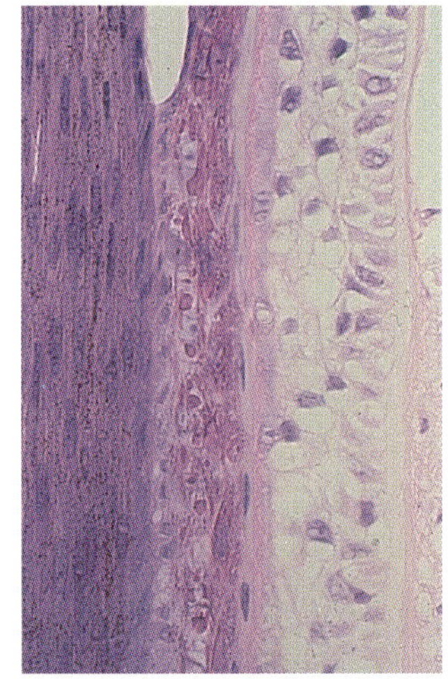

1.5b ■

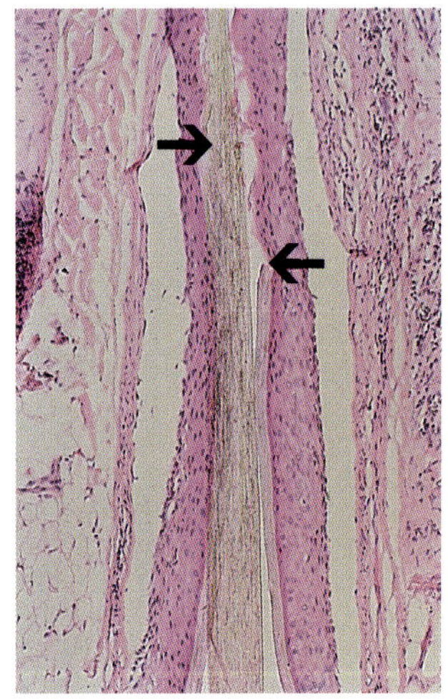

1.6

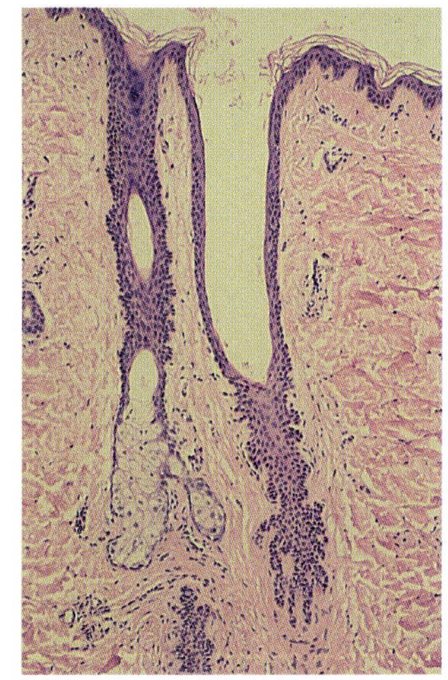

1.7

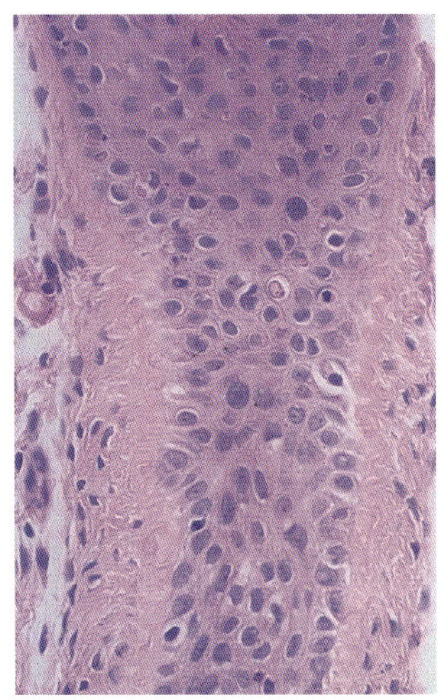

1.8

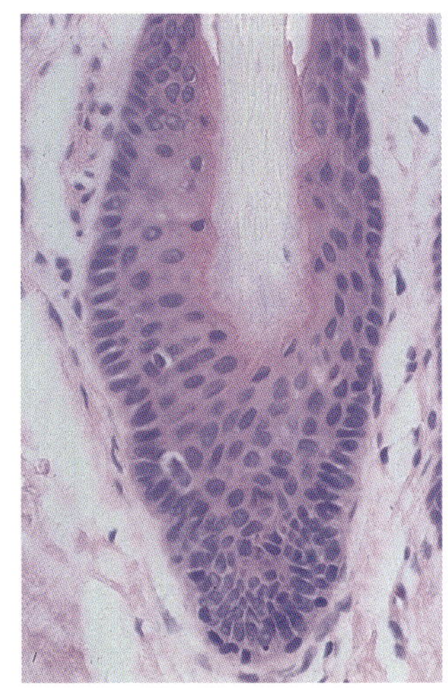

1.9

face epithelium which forms basket-weave keratin (Figure 1.7).

The embryological development of hair follicles begins by the end of the second month as an increased density of nuclei in the basal layer of the epidermis of the eyebrows, upper lip and chin, the areas where vibrissae form in other mammals. The initial population of hair follicle precursors is complete by 22 weeks' gestation. The growth of fine lanugo hair occurs and is shed by the end of the eighth month of gestation in a progressive wave from frontal to parietal areas. A second coat of lanugo hair appears and is shed in a more or less synchronized or wave pattern by the third or fourth month of life. The last hairs to enter telogen, usually after birth, are those over the occipital area. Eight to 12 weeks after entering telogen these hairs over the occipital area are lost and a definite patch of alopecia may appear.

By the end of the first year of life there is loss of synchronization. From this point the mosaic pattern, representing a random distribution of follicles in all stages of the growth cycle, is maintained.

The normal growth cycle of the individual follicle has been well defined. Anagen refers to the growth phase. It may be further divided into proanagen— those stages of anagen from development of a new hair until its emergence at the skin surface and metanagen—from emergence to onset of catagen. The average duration of anagen is approximately 1000 days (2 to 6 years). Catagen refers to the period of cessation of growth and is complete within a few weeks. Catagen is characterized by upward retraction of the hair shaft, thickening of the hyaline basement membrane, and individual cell necrosis or apoptosis of the outer root sheath or trichilemma (Figure 1.8). This hair displacement and volumetric reduction of trichilemma leads to the gradual disappearance of the transient, inferior segment of the follicle. Telogen refers to the resting phase which lasts approximately 100 days. The telogen hair is the resting or club hair with a nonpigmented bulb (Figure 1.9). It has retracted up the follicle to the lower end of the isthmus, represented by the bulge area of insertion of the arrector pili muscle. As a new anagen hair develops the club hair is shed and the cycle repeats itself.

The relative length of the phases of growth dictate that 5-10% of hairs are in the resting phase at any one time. Assuming that the average number of follicles in the human scalp equals 100,000, then up to 10,000 hairs could usually be expected to be in telogen at any one time. If telogen lasts 100 days, then an average daily loss of up to 100 hairs is not abnormal.

A dramatic change in current concepts of hair growth is an entirely new theory as to the source of germinal cells for the new anagen hair. Until recently it has been accepted that these stem cells originate in the hair bulb, but there is evidence to suggest that the bulge area of arrector pili muscle insertion at mid-follicular level is the site of stem cell origin. ■

Suggested Reading

Abell, E.: "Embyrology and anatomy of the hair follicle." In: *Disorders of Hair Growth. Diagnosis and Treatment,* Olsen, E.A. (Ed.). New York: McGraw–Hill 1994:1–19.

Ackerman, A.B., deViragh, P.A., Chongchitnant, N.: *Neoplasms with Follicular Differentiation.* Philadelphia: Lea and Febiger, 1993:21–102.

Bertolino, A.P., O'Guin, W.M.: "Differentiation of the hair shaft." In: *Disorders of Hair Growth. Diagnosis and Treatment,* Olsen, E.A. (Ed.). New York: McGraw–Hill 1994:21–37.

Champion, R.H., Gillman, T., Rook A., et al.: *An Introduction to the Biology of the Skin.* Oxford: Blackwell Scientific Publications, 1970:164–174.

Ebling, F.J.: "Biology of hair follicles." In: *Dermatology in General Medicine,* 3rd ed. Fitzpatrick, T.B., et al (Eds.). New York: McGraw Hill, 1987:213–219.

Jakubovic, H.R., Ackerman, A.B.: "Structure and function of skin: Development, morphology and physiology." In: *Dermatology,* (3rd ed.) Moschella, S.L., Hurley, H.J. (Eds.). Philadelphia: W.B. Saunders, 1992.

Jarrett, A., Ed.: *The Physiology and Pathophysiology of the Skin,* Vol. 4, The hair follicle. London: Academic Press, 1977:1237–1349.

Kligman, A.M.: "The human hair cycles." *J Invest Dermatol* 1959;33:307–316.

Messenger, A.G.: "Isolation, culture and in vitro behavior of cells isolated from the papilla of hair follicles." In: *Trends in Human Hair Growth and Alopecia Research* Van Neste D., Lachapelle, J.M., Antoine, J.L., (Eds.). Netherlands: Kluwer Academic 1989:57–67.

Messenger, A.G.: "The control of hair growth and pigmentation." In: *Disorders of Hair Growth. Diagnosis and Treatment,* Olsen, E.A. (Ed.). New York: McGraw–Hill 1994:39–58.

Miller, S.J., Sun, T–T, Lavker, R.M.: "Hair follicles, stem cells and skin cancer." *J Invest Dermatol* 1993;100:288S–294S.

Montagna, W., Parakkal, P.F.: *The Structure and Function of the Skin* (3rd Ed.). New York: Academic Press, 1974:172–258.

Orentreich, N.: "Scalp Hair Replacement in Man." In: Montagna, W., Dobson, R.L., Eds. *Advances in Biology of the Skin.* (Hair Growth, vol. 9). Oxford: Pergamon Press, 1969:99–108.

Philpott, M.P., Green, M.R., Kealey T.: "Human hair growth in vitro." *J Cell Sci* 1990;97:463–471.

Philpott, M.P., Green, M.R., Kealey, T.: "Rat hair follicle growth in vitro." *Br J Dermatol* 1992;127:600–607.

Rook, A., Wilkinson, D.S.,Ebling, F.J.G., et al.: *Textbook of Dermatology,* 4th ed. Oxford: Blackwell Scientific Publications, 1986:1937–2037.

Rook, A., Dawber, R.: *Diseases of the Hair and Scalp* (2nd ed.). Oxford: Blackwell Scientific Publications, 1991:1–48.

Weinberg, W.C., Goodman, L.V., George, C., et al.: "Reconstitution of hair follicle development in vivo: Determination of follicle formation, hair growth, and hair quality by dermal cells." *J Invest Dermatol* 1993;100:229–236.

Williams, R., Philpott, M.P., Kealey, T.: "Metabolism of freshly isolated human hair follicles capable of hair elongation. A glutaminolytic, aerobic, glycolytic tissue." *J Invest Dermatol* 1993;100:834–840.

Assessment of Patient with Hair Loss

Causes of Alopecia

From a practical standpoint it is useful to consider the causes of alopecia in decreasing order of frequency. The conditions listed here reflect experience at a dermatologic hair clinic, which may differ from that in a primary care setting:

- Androgenetic alopecia
- Diffuse alopecia
- Alopecia areata
- Cicatricial alopecia
- Traumatic alopecia
- Infections and infestations
- Abnormalities of the hair shaft causing alopecia
- Hereditary and congenital alopecia
- Miscellaneous causes of alopecia

The following systematic approach may be helpful in identifying the many different types and causes of alopecia.

Patient History

A detailed history should be taken in the evaluation of hair loss. Beware of making a snap diagnosis, as appearances may be deceptive and emotional overtones may need attention. The patient should be asked to complete a written questionnaire. The questionnaire can then be used as the basis for additional specific questions and a full examination later. The duration of the present and previous episodes of hair loss should be established. Appropriate questions regarding scalp hair loss are listed in Table 2.1. Any hair loss from face or body should be recorded. Details of any related hirsutism, as well as disorders of hair texture, scalp, teeth, nails and skin, both past and present, should be obtained. A hair care history can be obtained using the questions listed in Table 2.2 . Information relating to any previous treatment of the alopecia should be recorded. Ask specific questions about atopic and autoimmune diseases and about symptoms possibly relating to thyroid disorders, anemia and virilization. Also inquire about recent stressful events, such as crash diets, febrile or severe illnesses, operations, childbirth, and mental stress. Record the menstrual history where relevant. A careful family history of hair loss, abnormal hair texture, scalp disorders and autoimmune diseases is important. Record all drugs taken within the last year. A drug history questionnaire is given in Table 2.3 but this is subject to change over time.

Examination

Coloring
Hair, skin and eye color should be recorded.

Hair and Scalp Assessment
Diagrams are useful for recording the location, pattern and extent of the hair loss. The pattern of hair loss has diagnostic significance. Hair loss involving the top of the scalp predominantly while sparing the back and most of the sides of the scalp indicates androgenetic alopecia. Male pattern androgenetic alopecia is characterized by bitemporal reces-

Table 2.1 Scalp hair loss: Questionnaire

Check if answer is yes

☐ Is baldness generalized	☐ or patchy?
☐ Is the hair coming out by the roots	☐ or breaking off?
☐ Is excess hair seen on pillows	☐ and/or shoulders?
☐ Is excess hair seen in comb or brush	☐ and/or sink or drain?
☐ Is hair thinning noticed by you	☐ and/or by others?
☐ Is the hair loss continuous	☐ or has it stopped?
☐ Is the rate of hair loss increasing	☐ or decreasing?
☐ Is hair regrowing all over	☐ or in patches?
☐ Is your daily hair loss less than 100 hairs	☐ or more than 100?

Table 2.2 Hair care history: Questionnaire

Check if answer is yes

☐ Did you shampoo your hair today	☐ or yesterday?
☐ Do you shampoo your hair daily	☐ or every 2 to 3 days?
☐ Do you shampoo your hair weekly	☐ or at other intervals?
☐ Do you use a conditioner	☐ and hair spray or mousse?
☐ Does your hair care include blow drying	☐ and backcombing/teasing?
☐ Does your hair care include braiding or ponytails	☐ and/or cornrowing?
☐ Do you use rubber bands	☐ and rollers?
☐ Do you use pomades	☐ and/or hot combing?
☐ Do you use straighteners	☐ or relaxers?
☐ Do you use permanent waves	☐ or permanent dyes?
☐ Do you use color rinses	☐ or bleaches?
☐ Do you have your hair processed at home	☐ or in the beauty/barber shop?

Table 2.3 Drug history: Questionnaire

Check if answer is yes

☐ Allopurinol	☐ Alpha receptor blockers	☐ Amiodarone
☐ Amoxapine	☐ Androgens	☐ Angiotensin converting enzyme inhibitors
☐ Anticancer drugs	☐ Anticoagulants	☐ Anticonvulsants
☐ Antithyroid drugs	☐ Aspirin	☐ Azathioprine
☐ Azulfidine	☐ Beta blockers	☐ Birth control drugs
☐ Boric acid	☐ Bromocriptine	☐ Calcium channel blockers
☐ Carbamazepine	☐ Cholesterol reducers	☐ Clomiphene
☐ Clonidine	☐ Colchicine	☐ Estrogen
☐ Ethambutol	☐ Ethionamide	☐ Fluoxetine
☐ Gentamycin	☐ Gold	☐ Haloperidol
☐ Histamine 2 blockers	☐ Levodopa	☐ Lithium
☐ Methyldopa	☐ Methysergide	☐ Metyrapone
☐ Nitrofurantoin	☐ NSAIDS*	☐ Omeprazole
☐ Para amino salicylic acid	☐ Penicillamine	☐ Prazosin
☐ Probenecid	☐ Pyridostigimne bromide	☐ Retinoids
☐ Retinal	☐ Sulfasalazine	☐ Terfenadine
☐ Tricyclic Antidepressants		

* NSAIDS = nonsteroidal anti-inflammatory drugs

sion of hair with balding over the vertex (Figure 2.1). Female pattern androgenetic alopecia is characterized by a roughly oval area of diffuse hair loss over the top of the scalp with an intact frontal hairline (Figure 2.2) and no obvious balding over the vertex. A diffuse hair loss which involves the hair on the back and sides of the scalp as well as the top indicates an underlying systemic factor causing generalized loss. Fluctuating bitemporal recession of hair may be a feature of diffuse alopecia associated with telogen effluvium (Figure 2.3). A patchy alopecia may indicate alopecia areata, tinea capitis or trichotillomania, (Figure 2.4), or one of the many causes of cicatricial alopecia. A marginal or peripheral alopecia usually indicates a traction alopecia (Figure 2.5) although sometimes it may be due to alopecia areata of the ophiasis type.

The scalp needs to be examined for erythema, scaling, infection, the presence or absence of follicular orifices, other follicular abnormalities, scarring, atrophy, and neoplastic change.

The hair must be examined carefully over the entire scalp both visually and manually. The hair and scalp should be felt and the hair manipulated in various ways as indicated:

Hair Density: Hair density can be judged by parting the hair with a comb in a coronal plane in different areas of the scalp and comparing the part with those seen in normal subjects (Figures 2.6a,b). A recent method of hair density grading has been introduced by Savin in which a sagittal center part is made over the vertex and the width of the part is estimated in a coronal plane over the mid vertex. This is a useful measure of hair loss in androgenetic alopecia and is graded from 1 to 8 according to the extent of involvement (Figures 2.7a,b,c,d,e,f,g,h). A grading of the density and thickness of the occipital (donor) hair is useful if hair transplantation is under consideration: Grade A hair is thick and dense, Grade D is thin and sparse, and Grades B and C are in-between.

Short Hairs: Short hairs are more easily displayed against a background of white or black felt on a card placed perpendicular to the scalp along a part in the hair (Figure 2.8). Short hairs are also easily seen by pulling a clump of hairs through a hole in a plastic sheet with a crochet hook. Short hairs may be miniaturized, broken off, cut short, or newly growing and tapered. The degree of pigmentation and the thickness of the hair shaft are useful in distinguishing vellus, intermediate and terminal short hairs.

Exclamation Point Hairs: Exclamation point hairs are usually 3-4 mm in length and have an expanded free end characteristic of trichorrhexis nodosa (Figure 2.9), although some are tapered. They frequently have

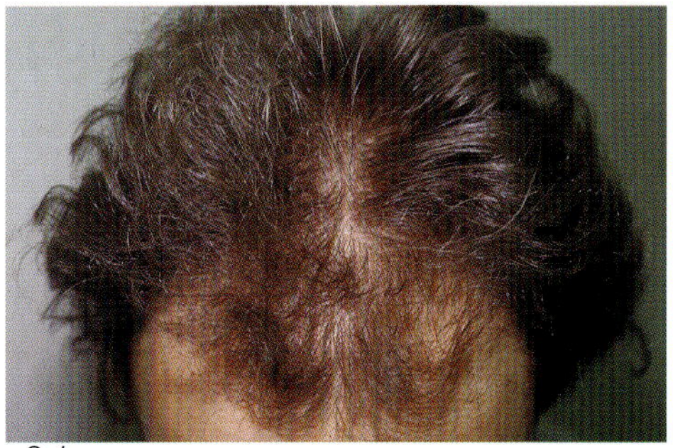
2.1

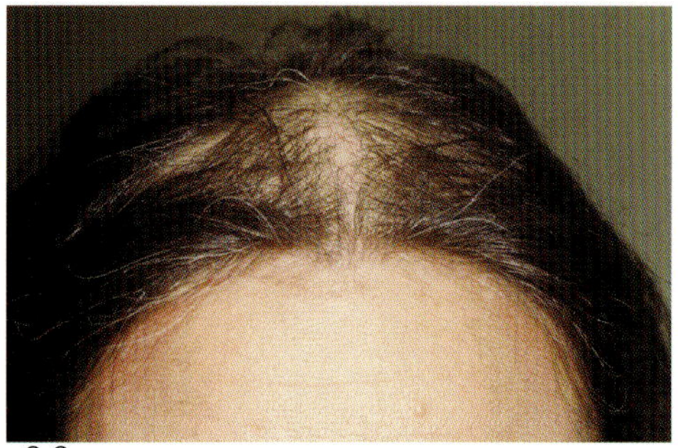
2.2

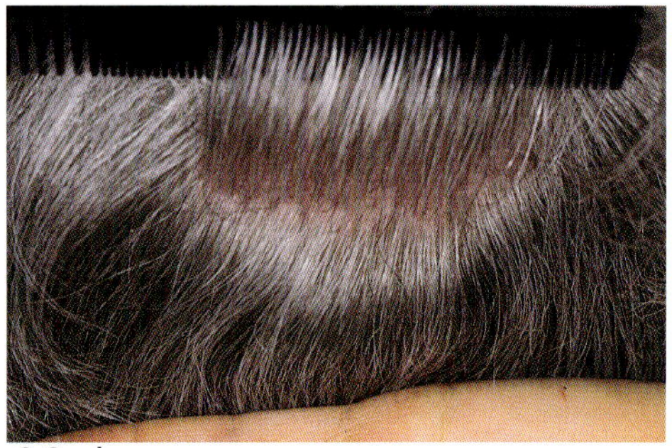
2.6a ↓

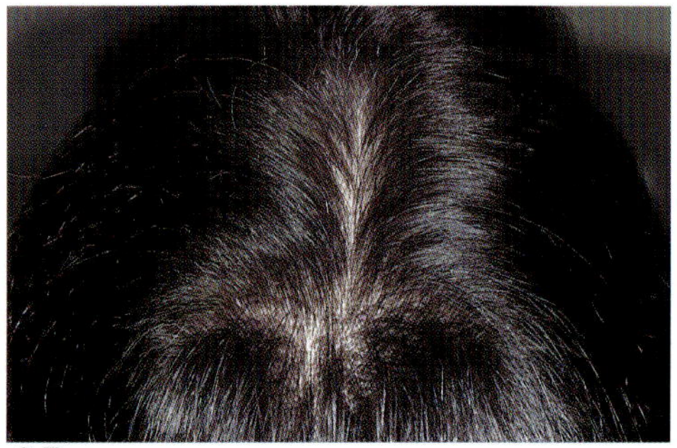
2.7a →

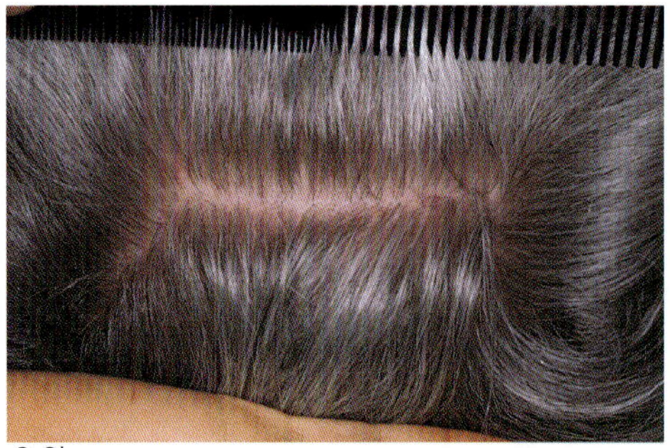
2.6b ■

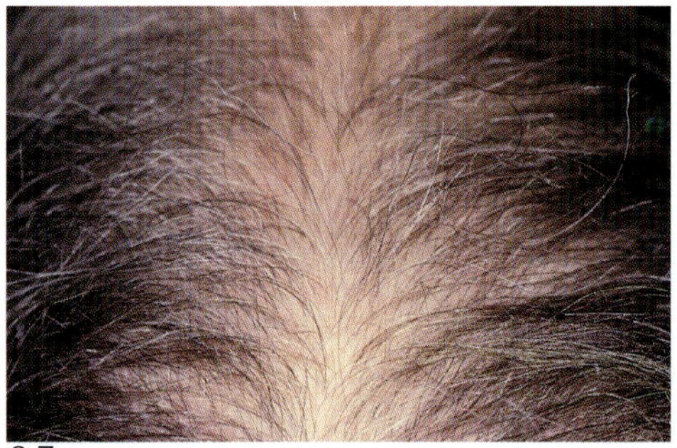
2.7e →

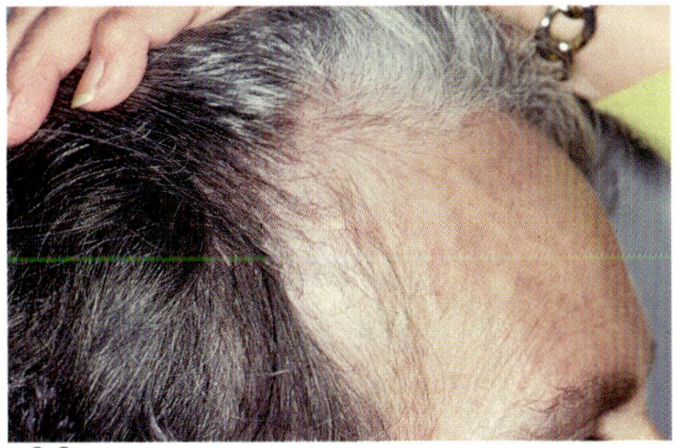
2.3

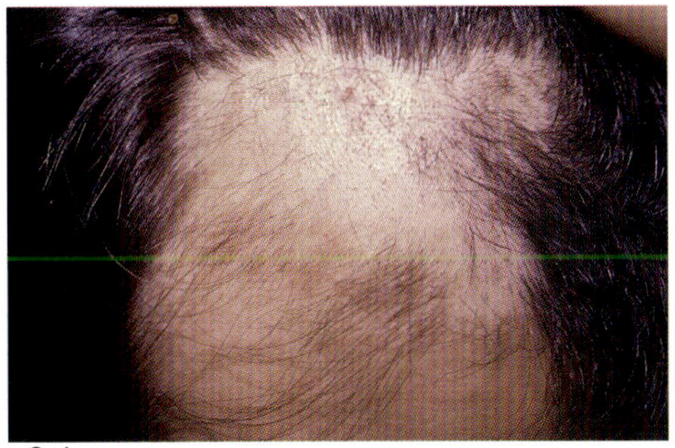
2.4

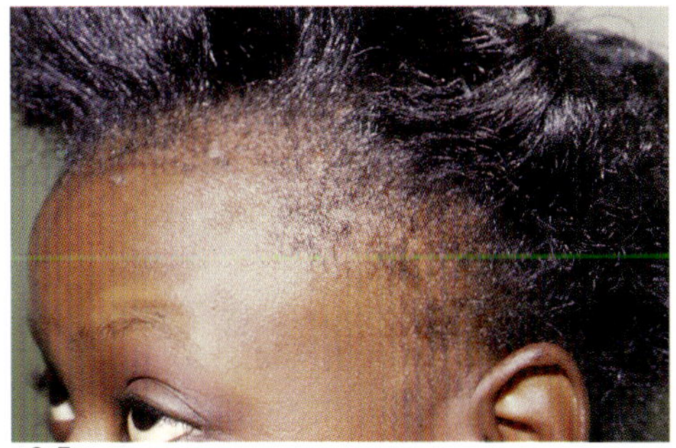
2.5

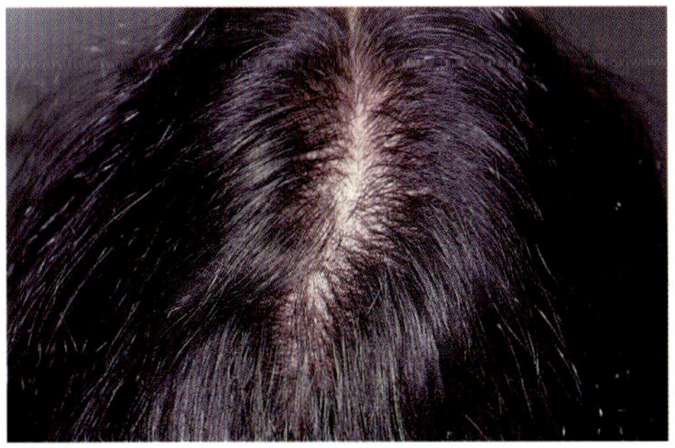
2.7b →

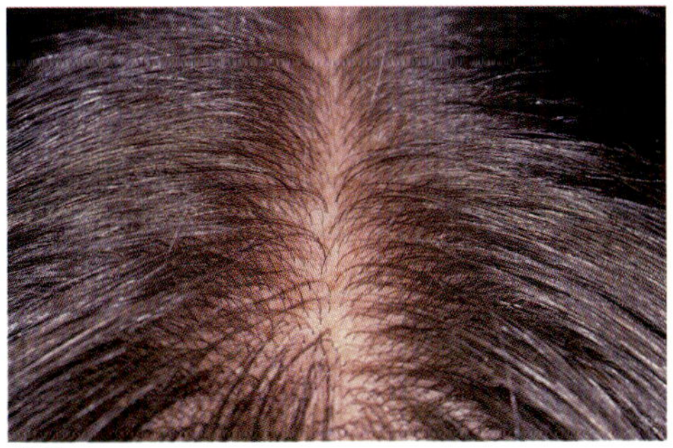
2.7c →

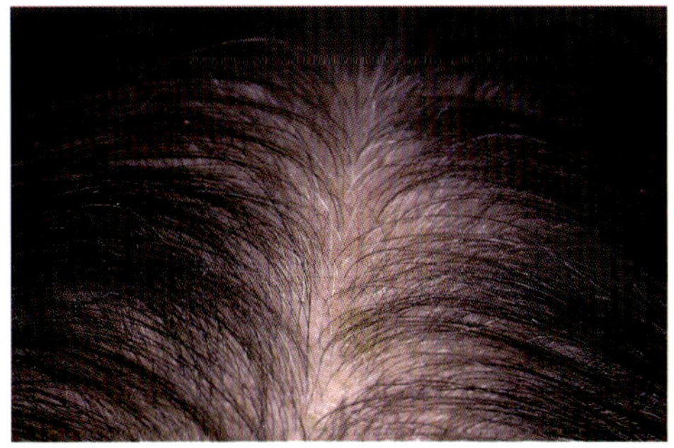
2.7d →

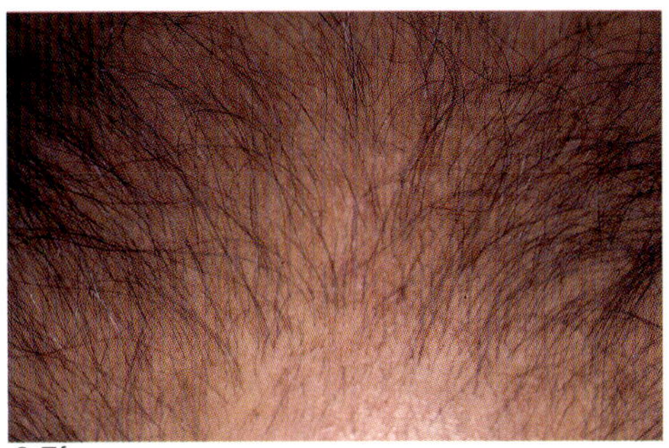
2.7f →

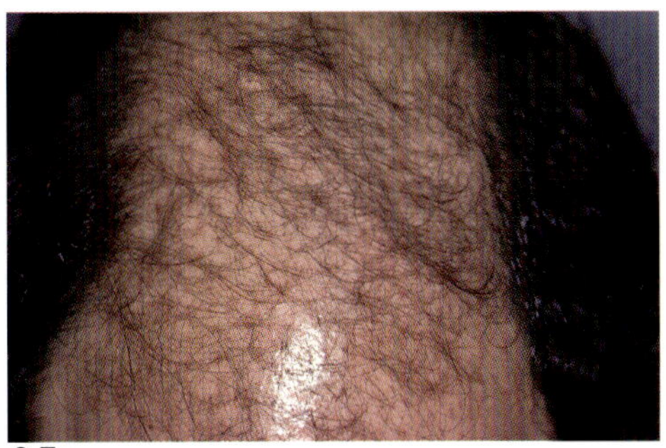
2.7g →

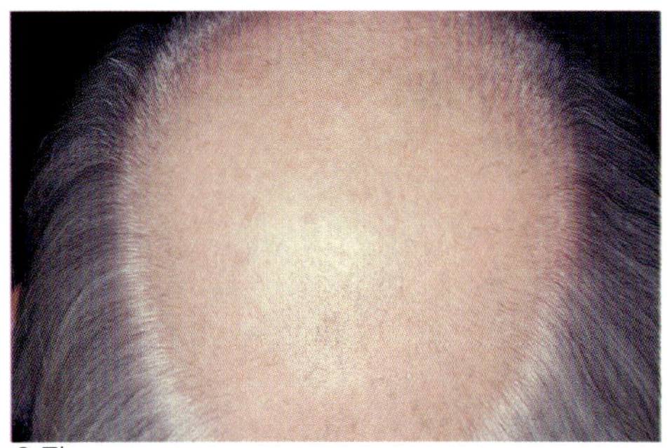
2.7h ■

2.1
Male pattern androgenetic alopecia: Hair loss from the frontal area and vertex, and hair recession in both temples.

2.2
Female pattern androgenetic alopecia: Central thinning of hair over the top of the scalp, with intact frontal margin and no bitemporal recession of hair.

2.3
Diffuse alopecia: Marked bitemporal recession of hair.

2.4
Patchy alopecia: The patchy hair loss is due to trichotillomania.

2.5
Marginal alopecia: The band of hair loss along the frontal hair margin is due to prolonged traction from hair styling.

2.6
Demonstration of hair density by hair part in coronal plane:

a. Normal density, shown by narrow hair part.

b. Widened hair part indicates reduced density of hair.

2.7
Mid vertex density scale *(after Savin, R.C. and the Upjohn Co. with permission)*:

a. Mid vertex density – Grade 1.

b. Mid vertex density – Grade 2.

c. Mid vertex density – Grade 3.

d. Mid vertex density – Grade 4.

e. Mid vertex density – Grade 5.

f. Mid vertex density – Grade 6.

g. Mid vertex density – Grade 7.

h. Mid vertex density – Grade 8.

depigmented, telogen roots but can have dystrophic, anagen roots. They occur characteristically along the spreading margins of patches of alopecia areata but may show a random scatter in cases of early diffuse alopecia areata.

Brittle Hair: Brittle hairs can be demonstrated by "feathering." In this technique the free distal ends of a group of hairs are gripped between thumb and forefinger and the fingers are then slid briskly towards the tips of the hair. Brittle hairs will leave short fragments on the fingers (Figure 2.10).

Hair Pull Tests: Hair pull tests should be done in different locations on the scalp. A group of 20 to 50 hairs is grasped securely at the base and pulled steadily but firmly outward toward the free ends of the hair. No more than one or two hairs out of every 10 grasped should normally detach. More than 2 of 10 hairs detaching is suggestive of increased hair loss (Figure 2.11). Usually the hairs that are pulled out in this way are telogen hairs with depigmented, club roots. Hair pull tests should be done on several different locations on the scalp so that the clinician becomes familiar with the technique. Normal hair pull tests will soon be recognized. Note that a recent shampoo will reduce the number of extractable hairs.

Hair Pluck Test: The hair pluck test is still used extensively by those who do routine trichograms, but has now lost popularity with many clinicians. It does allow direct anagen and telogen counts to be made, but counts of dystrophic hairs are unreliable since much of the observed hair dystrophy is artifactual due to hair damage caused by the plucking procedure itself. The test consists of forcible extraction of 40 or 50 hairs by a hemostat or needle holder (Figure 2.12). Some investigators favor the unit area trichogram in which a fixed area is marked on the scalp through a template and all the hairs in that area are individually epilated with tweezers and mounted on a slide for counting.

Hair Counts: Daily scalp hair counts may be useful in patients with diffuse alopecia which is inapparent to the observer. The patient is instructed to collect all hairs seen in the morning on the pillows, sheets, shoulders, brush and comb or in the sink and shower, using a net over the drain. These hairs are placed daily in separate plastic (sandwich) bags and labeled with the date and total hair count. Each shampoo day is indicated by an "S." Hair samples are collected over a two-week period. For most people an average daily loss of up to 100 hairs is normal, and in those with very thick hair an average loss of up to 150 hairs a day can be normal.

Test of Hair Growth: Hair growth can be tested using the so-called "hair growth window" technique. A measured 1 cm square patch on the vertex is shaved flush with the scalp and covered by an occlusive patch

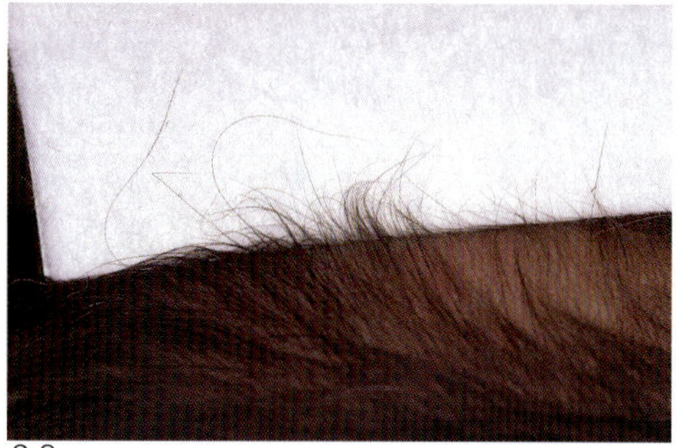

2.8

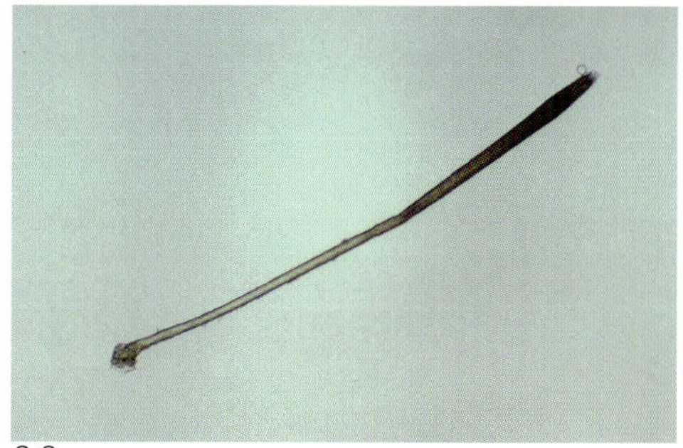

2.9

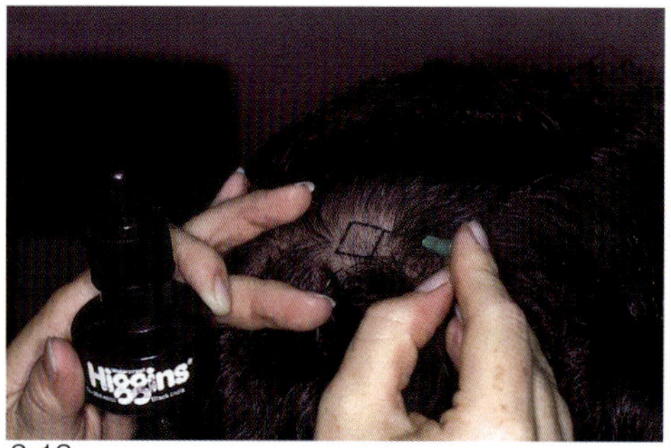

2.13

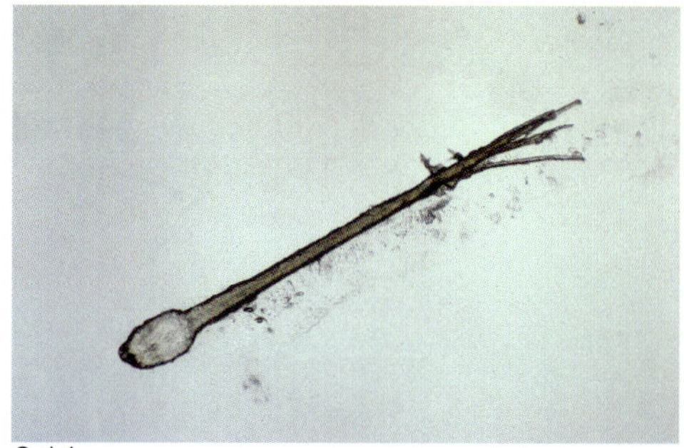

2.14

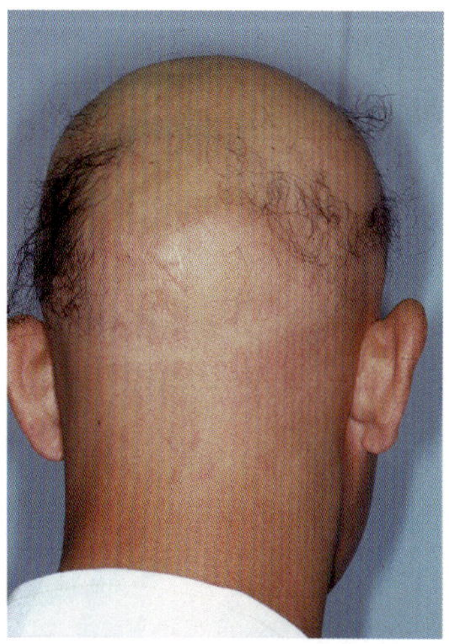

2.15a →

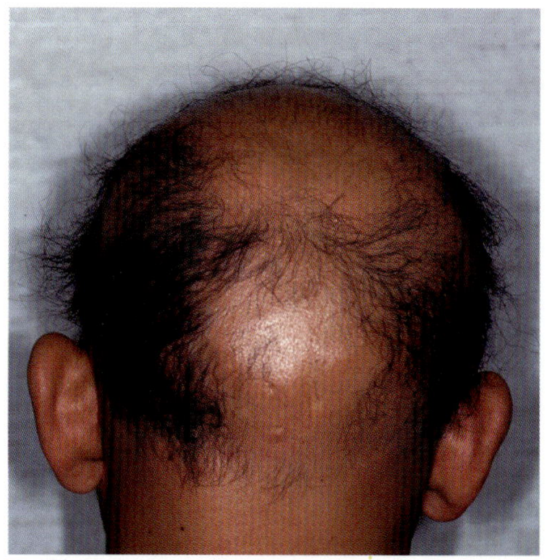

2.15b ■

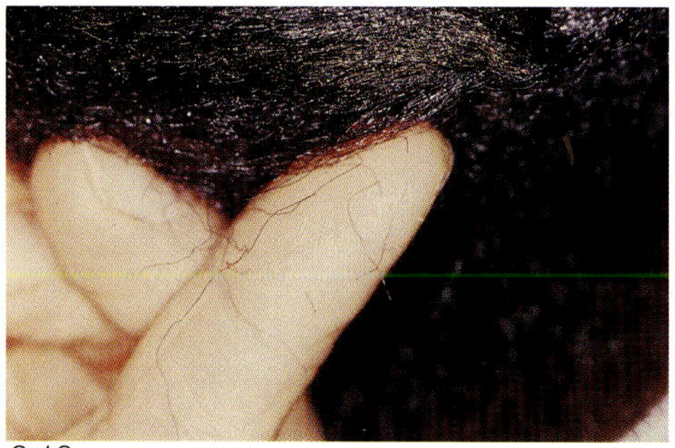

2.10

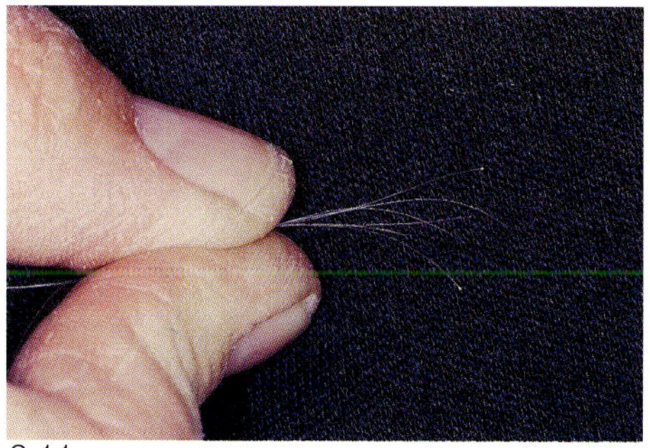

2.11

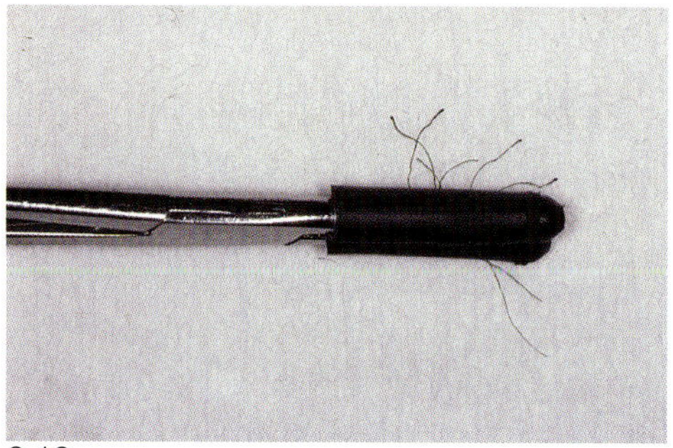

2.12

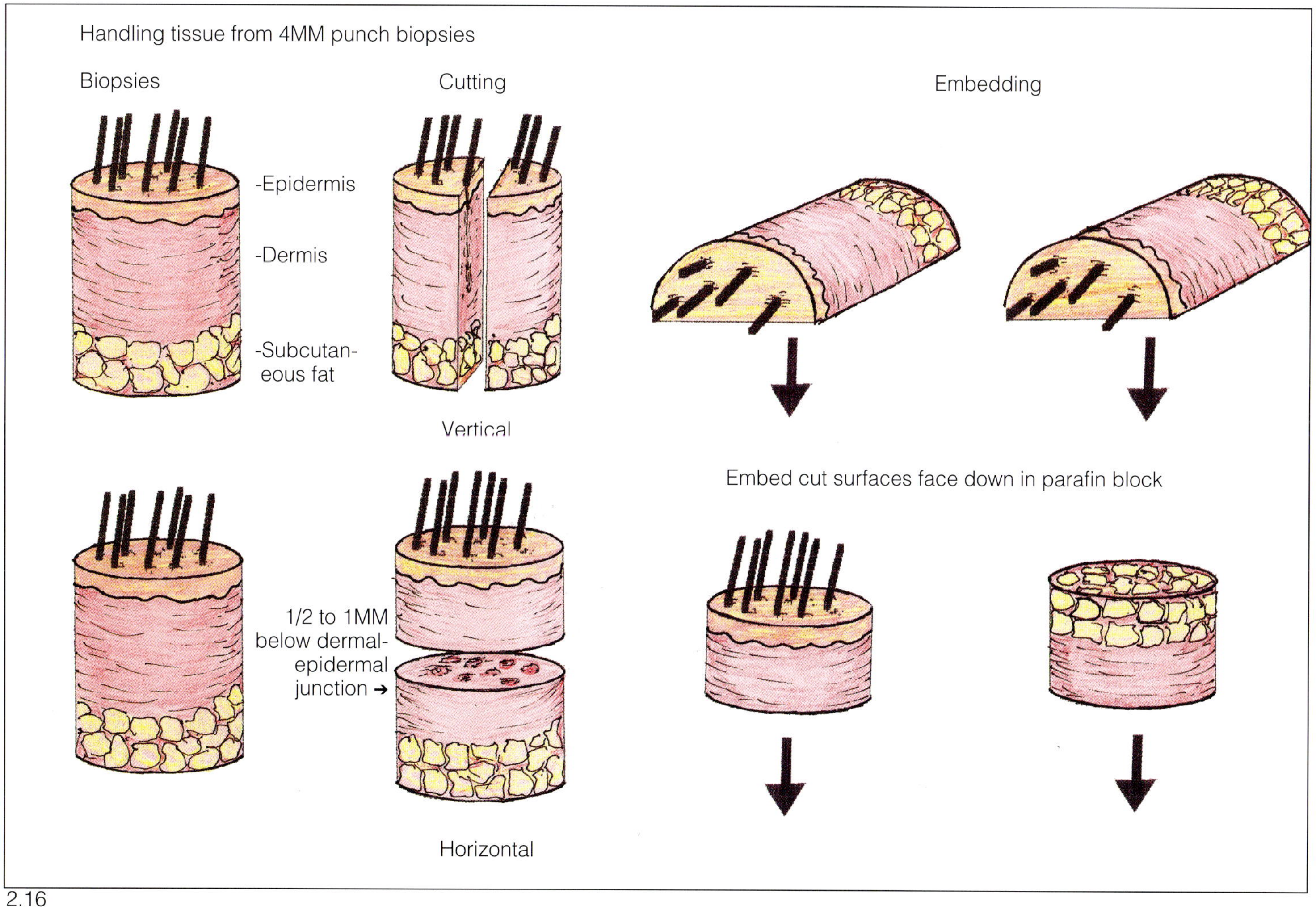

2.16

2.8
Demonstration of newly growing anagen hairs: Dark hairs stand out against a white card placed across scalp in coronal plane.

2.9
Exclamation point hair: Hair removed from active patch of alopecia areata shows a club root and a transverse fracture from trichorrhexis nodosa at the distal end. LM x 40.

2.10
Hair feathering: Short fragments of brittle hair are visible on the fingers with this technique.

2.11
Hair pull test: This group of 5 hairs, detached from 10 or 12 hairs grasped on the scalp, indicates a positive test.

2.12
Hair pluck test: This is carried out by forcible extraction of a group of hairs by a rubber–tipped hemostat or needle holder.

2.13
Hair growth window: A 1 cm square patch of hair is shaved, marked and occluded for a week or two, after which new hair growth is measured.

2.14
Light microscopy: Telogen hair with club root and frayed distal end, or trichoptilosis, caused by trichotillomania. LM x 40.

2.15
Clinical photography:

a. Alopecia areata before treatment.

b. Alopecia areata after treatment.

2.16
Scalp biopsy: Diagram of method used for cutting and embedding vertical and horizontal sections of scalp biopsies.

2.17
Scalp biopsy: Vertical section: Terminal hairs: Hair follicles are rooted in the subcutaneous tissue. LM x 40.

2.18
Scalp biopsy: Horizontal sections: Terminal anagen hair: Hair bulb:

a. Lower portion: Dermal papilla. LM x 400.

b. Upper portion: Matrix. LM x 400.

2.19
Scalp biopsy: Horizontal sections: Terminal anagen hair: Inferior segment of follicle:

a. Keratinizing inner root sheath in vicinity of hair bulb. LM x 400.

b. Henley's layer is the first to keratinize in the inner root sheath, followed by the cuticle of the inner root sheath. LM x 400.

c. Huxley's layer is the last to keratinize in the inner root sheath. LM x 400.

d. Keratinization of the inner root sheath is complete, mid way up the inferior segment of the follicle. LM x 400.

2.20
Scalp biopsy: Horizontal sections: Terminal hair: Isthmus and infundibulum:

a. Isthmus: Inner root sheath is being replaced by trichilemmal keratin. LM x 400.

b. Infundibulum: Terminal hairs are surrounded by loose keratin. LM x 100.

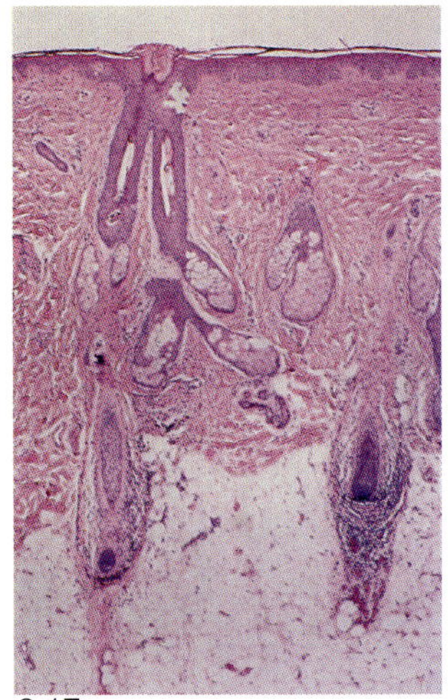
2.17

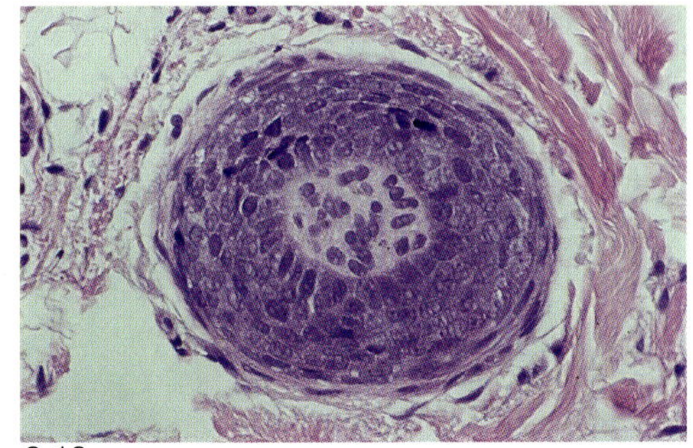
2.18a →

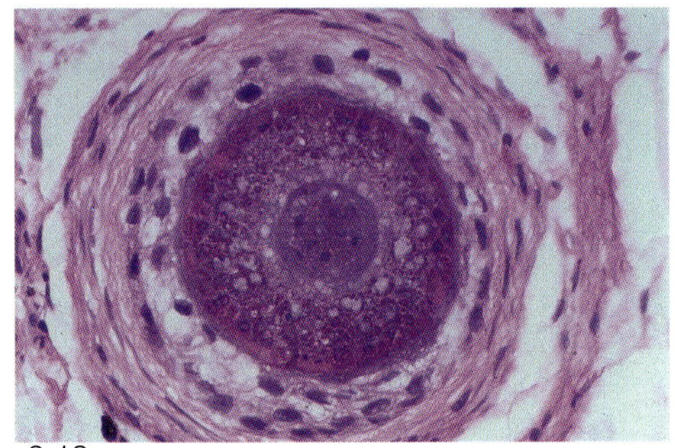
2.19a →

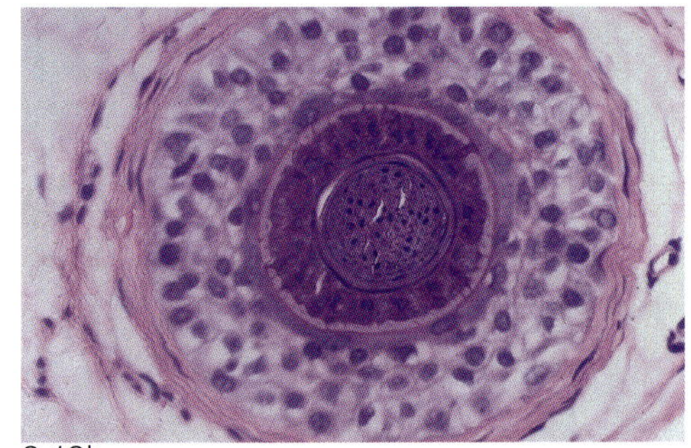
2.19b →

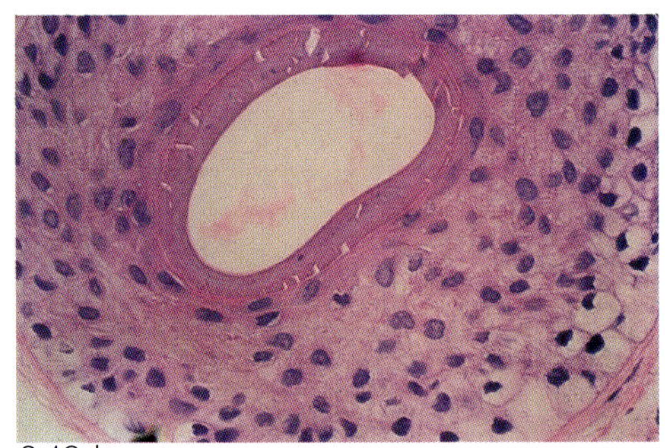
2.19d ■

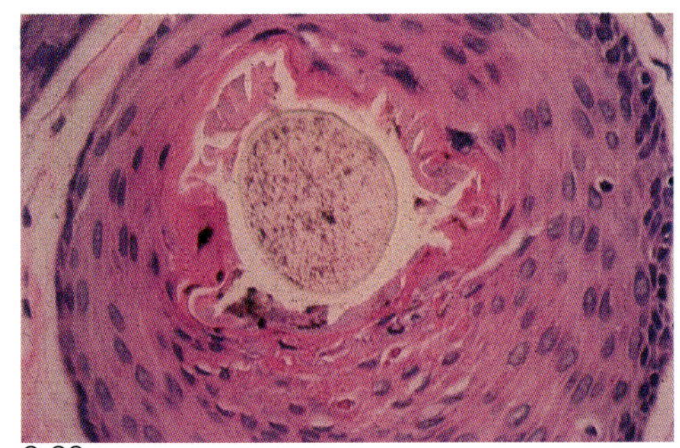
2.20a →

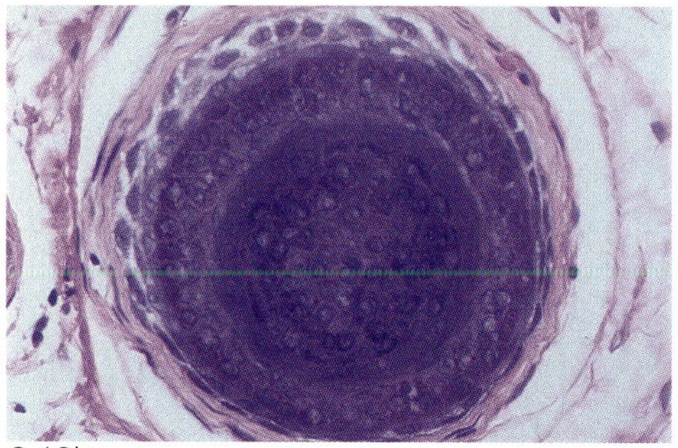

2.18b ■

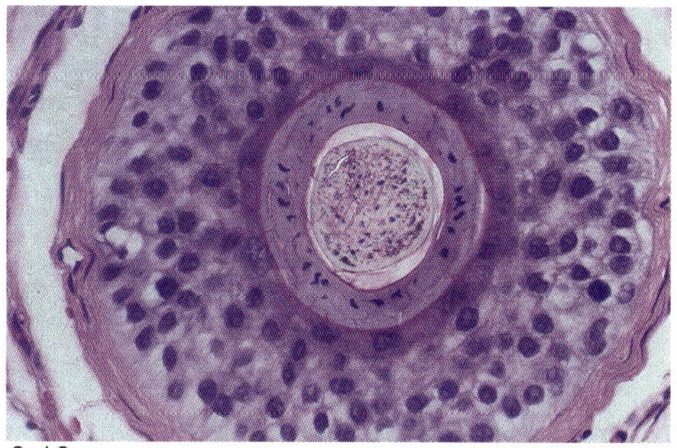

2.19c ➔

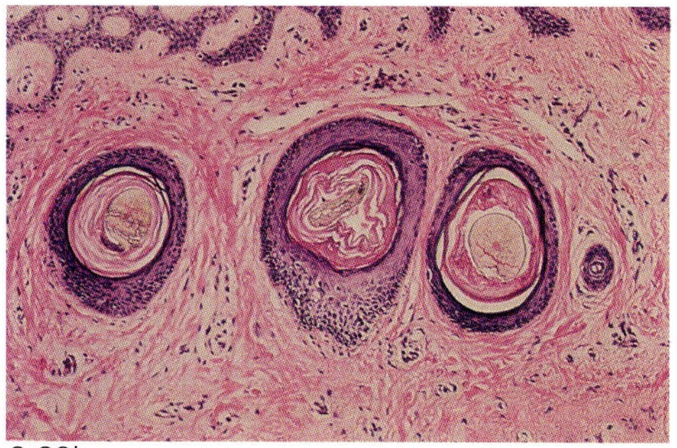

2.20b ■

for 1 to 2 weeks. The patch is then removed, and the length of the recently cut hairs is measured (Figure 2.13). Weekly growth of 2.5 mm is normal.

Light Microscopy: Light microscopic examination of hair is often required. It is best to examine hairs with intact roots, preferably after they have been extracted as gently as possible with the fingers (Figure 2.14). Hair shafts can be examined in hairs that have been cut off flush with the scalp using sharp scissors. Individual hairs should be mounted in parallel either between two glass slides taped together at the ends or on glass slides previously coated with double-stick clear tape or two fresh bands of mounting medium. In making permanent preparations hairs should be placed in parallel on the glass slide and a long cover slip applied using mounting medium. Roots should be examined to determine the stage of the hair cycle and for the presence of dystrophy. The hair shafts should be examined to detect fractures, irregularities, coiling and twisting, and extraneous matter. The free ends of the hair should be checked to see whether they are tapered, cut, fractured, or weathered. If fungal diseases are suspected, hairs should be placed on a glass slide with 20% potassium hydroxide added in order to demonstrate fungal spores and hyphae.

Scanning Electron Microscopy: Scanning electron microscopy is generally used as a research tool and is usually not required for diagnostic purposes. There are some hair shaft abnormalities such as uncombable hair with longitudinal grooving which are better seen with scanning electron microscopy.

Photography: Photography is useful for record purposes (Figures 2.15a,b). However, photographs can be misleading due to changes in hair styling.

Scalp Biopsies: Scalp biopsies are indicated in all cases of cicatricial alopecia and in all cases of unexplained alopecia. It is traditional for skin biopsies to be cut in a vertical plane with the epidermis at the top and the subcutaneous tissue at the bottom. Most clinicians prefer to limit their scalp biopsies to 4 mm diameter punches which are sometimes inadequate for diagnostic purposes. It is useful to take two 4 mm punch biopsies from comparable sites of alopecia and section one vertically and the other horizontally (Figures 2.16, 2.17). If necessary, one half of the biopsy sectioned vertically can be used for immunofluorescence. In the horizontal sections, all follicular structures including hair bulbs, terminal anagen, catagen and telogen hairs, telogen germinal units, "vellus" hairs, follicular units and follicular stelae (streamers) are counted (Figures 2.18a,b, 2.19a,b,c,d 2.20a,b, 2.21a,b, 2.22a,b,c,d). The ratios of terminal to "vellus" and velluslike hairs, and of anagen to telogen hairs, are easily derived from these counts. Dividing the total hair count by 13 gives the concentration of hairs/mm^2 in a 4 mm punch biopsy cut horizontally. The concentration of follicular structures per unit area can give useful diagnostic information as well as predictive information regarding the possiblity of future regrowth (Table 2.4). Inflammatory changes, fibrosis and any visible epidermal changes are also noted.

Transmission Electron Microscopy: Transmission electron microscropy of scalp biopsy material is not a necessity for diagnostic purposes, but may be of considerable value in research.

Systemic Assessment

Systemic assessment should include the vital signs of weight, pulse, blood pressure, and a general examination made for signs of anemia, thyroid disorder and virilization. The nails and teeth should also be examined.

Laboratory Tests

A basic laboratory workup should include a complete blood count, routine chemistry studies, urinalysis, a serological test for syphilis, and tests of thyroid function as well as serum iron and ferritin levels. If indicated, tests of androgenic function might include determination of the serum levels of total testosterone, sex hormone binding globulin, dihydroepiandrosterone sulfate, androstenedione, and 3a, 17B–androstenediol glucuronide. Where additional tests of sex hormones status are required, serum levels of luteinizing hormone, follicle-stimulating hormone, and prolactin can be measured. Other tests should be done when indicated.

(continued)

Diagnosis

The diagnosis depends upon a combination of findings obtained from the history, physical examination and any necessary investigations. The differential diagnosis of alopecia will be considered in descending order of frequency in subsequent sections. ■

2.21
Scalp biopsy: Horizontal sections: Terminal hair: Inferior segment of hair follicle:

a. Terminal catagen hair: Trichilemma is being reduced in volume by apoptosis, and is surrounded by thickened, hyaline, basement membrane. LM x 400.

b. Terminal telogen or club hair: Central star-shaped area of trichilemmal keratin is surrounded by trichilemma. The outer cells show palisading. Apotosis is not seen and thickening of the hyaline membrane is no longer pronounced. LM x 400.

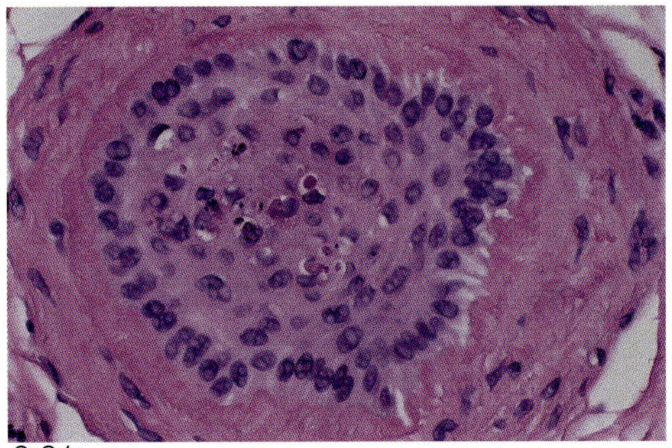

2.21a →

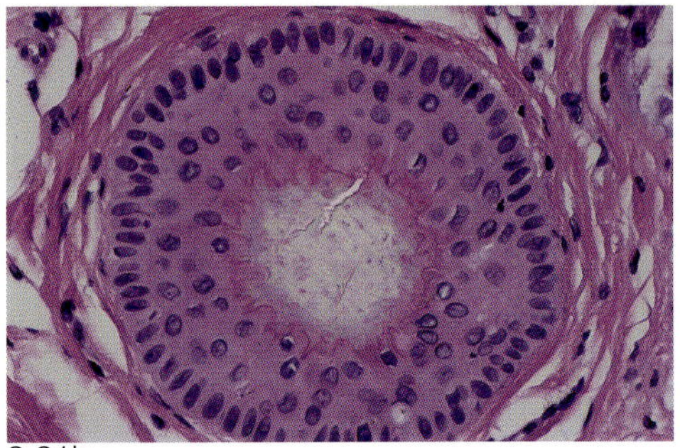

2.21b ■

2.22
Scalp biopsy: Horizontal sections:

a. Telogen germinal unit (mid follicular level): This irregular island of basoloid cells with peripheral palisading represents the resting hair follicle. LM x 400.

b. Vellus hair (papillary dermis level): A "vellus" hair is defined as a hair with a diameter that does not exceed 0.03 mm and that is smaller than the diameter of the investing root sheath. LM x 400.

c. Follicular units (mid follicular level of entry of sebaceous duct): Each hexagonal follicular unit encloses sebaceous glands, sebaceous ducts, and several terminal and/or "vellus" hairs. LM x 40.

d. Follicular stelae (level of reticular dermis or subcutaneous tissue): Each stela or streamer indicates pathway of the ascending hair follicle as it passes into a telogen phase or as it miniaturizes in androgenetic alopecia or alopecia areata. The stela is represented by an angiofibrotic whorl. LM x 400.

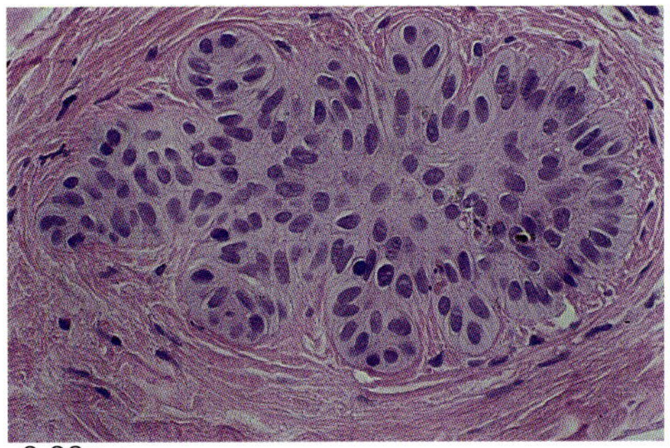

2.22a →

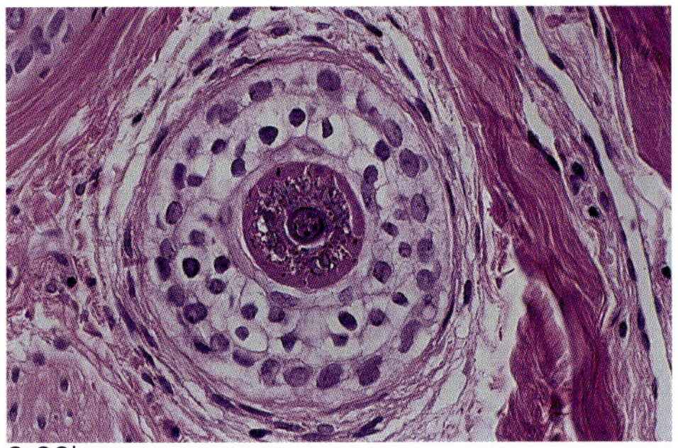

2.22b →

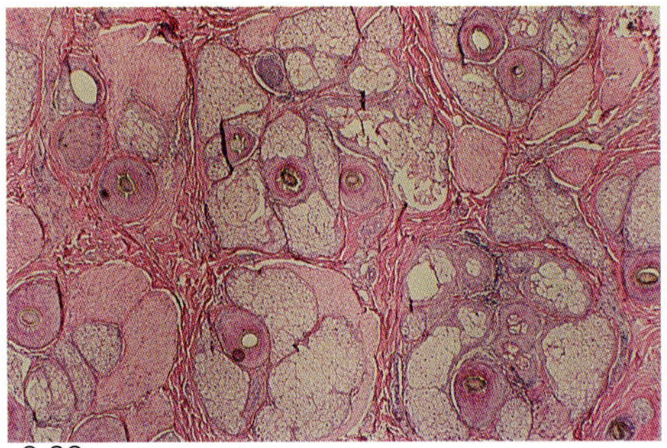

2.22c →

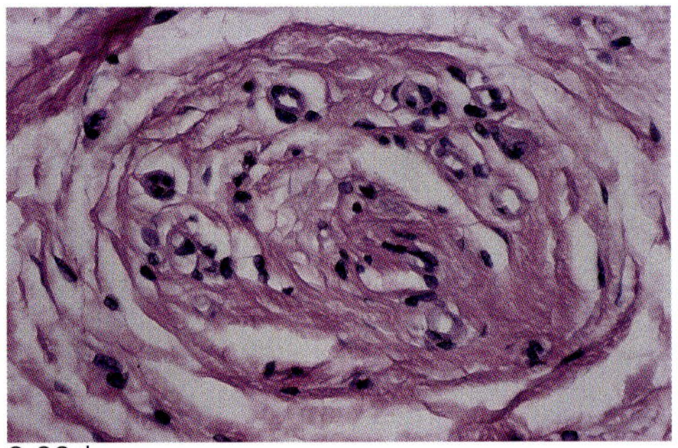

2.22d ■

Table 2.4 Horizontal Sections of 4mm–Diameter Punch Biopsies of Scalp

Follicular Counts in Differential Diagnosis of Alopecia*

Diagnosis	No. of Patients	Age	Sex M:F	Terminal(T) Hairs	+ Vellus(V) Hairs**	Total Hairs	T:V Ratio	Anagen:Telogen Ratio %
Normal controls	22	43	1.4:1	35	+ 5	=40	7:1	93.5:6.5
Androgenetic alopecia	412	40	1:1.1	23	+12	=35	1.9:1	83:17
Chronic telogen effluvium	355	44	1:38	35	+ 4	=39	9:1	89:11
Alopecia areata	290	32	1:1.7	14	+13	=27	1.1:1	73:27
Trichotillomania	34	22	1:5	32	+ 7	= 39	5:1	58:42

*After Whiting, D.A. Horizontal sections of scalp biopsies. In Dermatology: Progress and Perspectives. New York: Parthenon Publishing Group, 1993:215–216.
**Vellus (V) hairs include velluslike hairs with hairshaft diameter less than 0-.03mm.

Suggested Reading

Baden, H.P.: *Diseases of the hair and nails.* Chicago: Year Book Medical Publishers, Inc., 1987:115–120.

Braun–Falco, O., Heilgemeir, G.P.: "The Trichogram." *Semin Dermatol* 1985;4:40–52.

Ebling, F.J.G., Dawber, R., Rook, A.: "Differential diagnosis of alopecia." In: Rook, A., Wilkinson, D.S., Ebling, F.J.G., Champion, R.H., Burton, R.L., Eds.: *Textbook of Dermatology. 4th Ed.* Oxford: Blackwell Scientific Publications, 1986;3:2018– 2020.

Eckert, J., Church, R.E., Ebling, F.J.: "The pathogenesis of alopecia areata." *Br J Dermatol* 1968;80:203–210.

Headington, J.T.: "Transverse microscopic anatomy of the human scalp: a basis for a morphometric approach to disorders of the hair follicle." *Arch Dermatol* 1984;120:449–456.

Hordinsky, M.K.: "General evalution of the patient with alopecia." *Dermatol Clin* 1987;5:483–489.

Modly, C.E., Wood, C.M., Burnett, J.W.: "Evaluation of alopecia: a new algorithm." *Cutis* 1989;43:148–152.

Olsen, E.A.: "Clinical tools for assessing hair loss." *In: Disorders of Hair Growth. Diagnosis and Treatment,* Olsen, E.A. (Ed.). New York: McGraw–Hill 1994, 59–69.

Pariser, D.M., Caserio, R.J., Eaglestein, W.H.: *Techniques for Diagnosing Skin and Hair Disease, 2nd ed.* New York: Thieme, 1986:143–179.

Price, V.H.:"Disorders of the hair in children." *Pediatr Clin North Amer* 1975;25:305– 320.

Rushton, H., James, K.C., Mortimer, C.H.: "The unit area trichogram in the assessment of androgen–dependent alopecia." *Br J Dermatol* 1983;109:429–437.

Savin, R.C.: "A method for visually describing hair loss in both male and female androgen alopecia." *Poster exhibit #23,24. 51st Annual Meeting, American Academy of Dermatology.* San Francisco,1992.

Shelley, W.B.: "Hair examination using double–stick tape." *J Am Acad Dermatol* 1983;8:430–431. (Letter to Editor).

Sperling, L.C., Heiner II, W.L.: "Androgen biology as a basis for the diagnosis and treatment of androgenic disorders in women." *I. J Am Acad Dermatol* 1993;28:669– 683.

Sperling, L.C., Heiner II, W.L.: "Androgen biology as a basis for the diagnosis and treatment of androgenic disorders in women." *II. J Am Acad Dermatol* 1993;28:901–916.

Stroud, J.D.: "Diagnosis and management of the hair loss patient." *Cutis* 1987;40:272–276.

Whiting, D.A.: "The Diagnosis of Alopecia." *Current Concepts,* Kalamazoo: The Upjohn Co., 1990.

Whiting, D.A.: "Structural abnormalities of the hair shaft." *J Am Acad Dermatol* 1987;16:1–25.

Whiting, D.A.: "Horizontal sections of scalp biopsies." In Burgdorf, W.H.C., Katz, S.I., Eds: *Dermatology: Progress and Perspectives.* The Proceedings of the 18th World Congress of Dermatology, New York, June 12-18, 1992. New York: Parthenon Publishing Group, 1993:215–216.

Whiting, D.A.: "The value of horizontal sections of scalp biopsies." *J Cutan Aging Cosmet Dermatol* 1990;1:165–173.

Whiting, D.A.: "Diagnostic and predictive value of horizontal sections of scalp biopsy specimens in male pattern androgenetic alopecia." J AM Acad Dermatol 1993; 28:755-763.

Androgenetic Alopecia

Definition

Androgenetic alopecia (AGA) is the common type of nonscarring hair loss affecting the crown which results from a genetically determined end-organ sensitivity to androgens. It is often referred to as simple baldness, male-pattern and female-pattern alopecia, hereditary alopecia, diffuse alopecia and baldness.

Etiology

Hair follicles in the temples, frontal region and vertex are genetically programed to revert from terminal to velluslike ("vellus") follicles when continuously exposed to androgens. This is seen as a progressive miniaturization of hair follicles from terminal through intermediate to "vellus." There is a concomitant shortening of the anagen cycle and a resultant increase in the proportion of telogen hairs. The timing and extent of baldness represents a complex interaction between genetic information and androgen metabolism. The genetic pattern is considered to be autosomal dominant with variable penetrance.

Clinical Description

In androgenetic alopecia thinning occurs without scaling or subjective symptoms predominantly on the top of the scalp with sparing of the back and sides of the scalp. In a young patient the complaint of increased hair loss often precedes the appearance of alopecia. The presence of a family history of alopecia should be established.

Male–Pattern Alopecia

In males thinning may begin at any time after puberty and is not unusual by the late teens. The incidence of alopecia increases with the age studied. As a rule of thumb 25% of men aged 25, 40% of men aged 40, and 50% of men aged 50 show evidence of androgenetic alopecia. Extensive efforts to classify both type and extent of common baldness have resulted in the modified Hamilton scale. The two components of male pattern baldness are bitemporal recession and balding over the vertex. Usually the balding starts in the temples and frontal areas and involves the posterior vertex later; occasionally the whole crown is affected by the thinning process from the start. The hair loss process may be gradual and continuous, but is often episodic. As the condition progresses, more of the vertex is involved by the balding process and in the most extreme cases complete balding of the crown can result, with hair remaining only on the back and sides of the scalp (Figures 3.1a,b,c,d,e,f,g).

(continued)

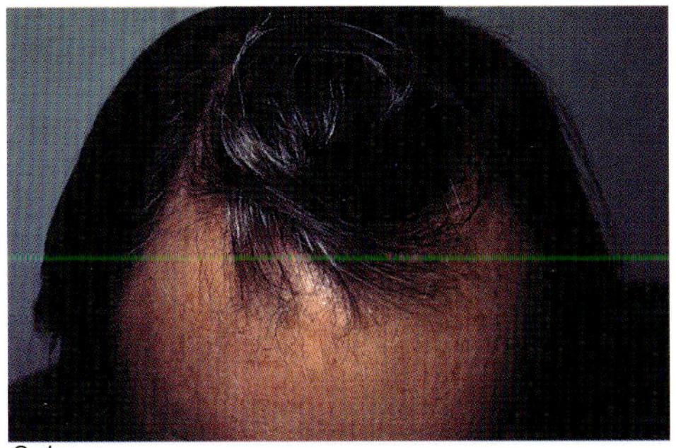

3.1a →

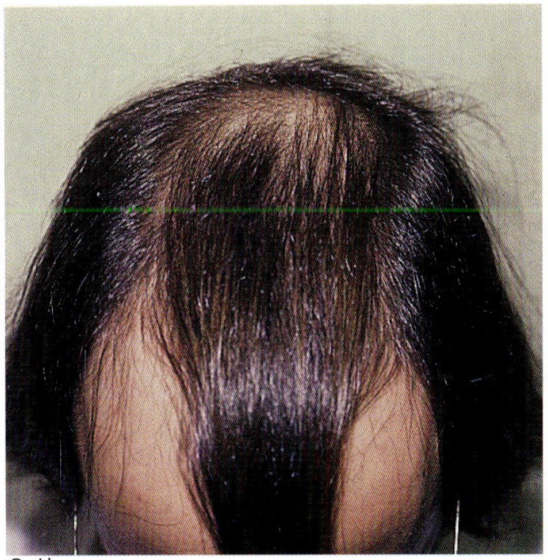

3.1b →

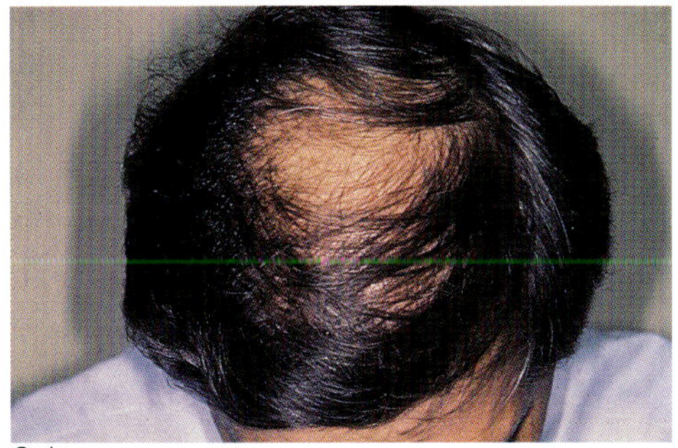

3.1c →

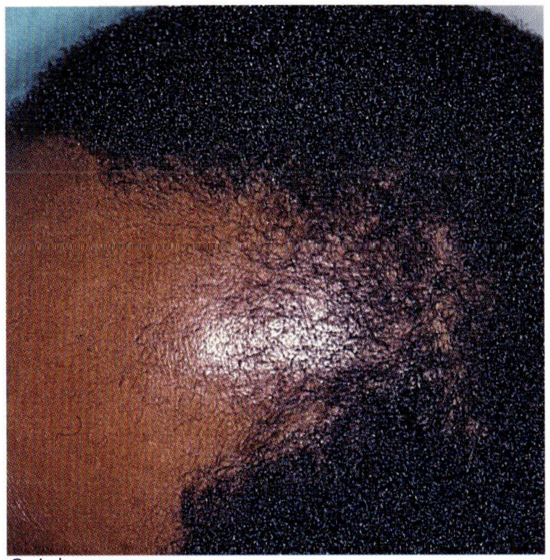

3.1d →

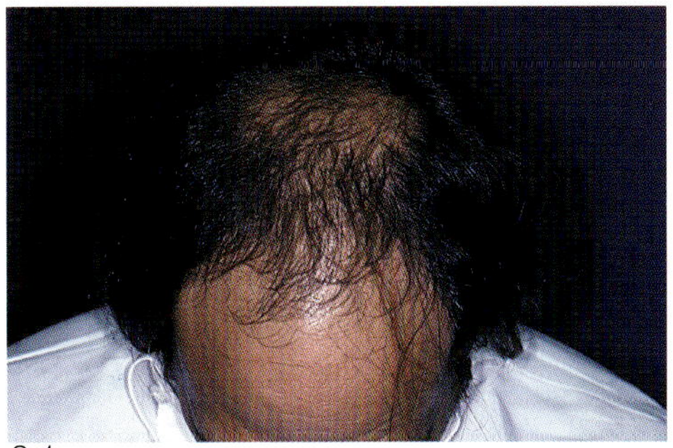

3.1e →

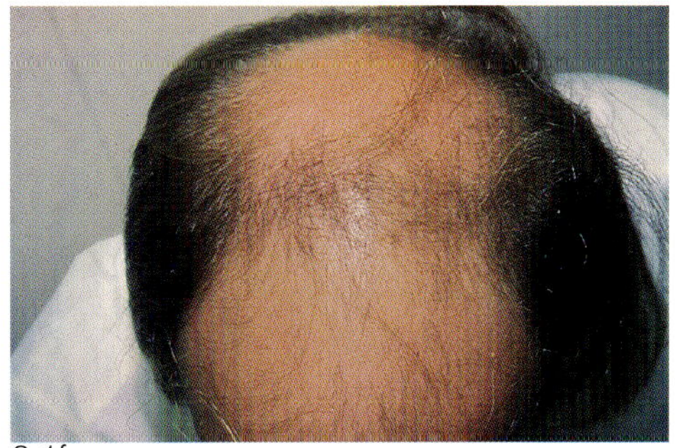

3.1f →

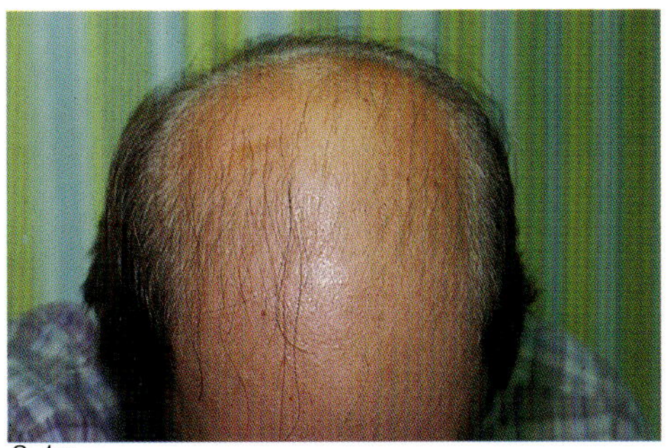

3.1g ■

3.1
Male androgenetic alopecia (AGA): Hamilton–Norwood classification:

a. Type III male AGA with bitemporal recession of hair.

b. Type III vertex male AGA with bitemporal recession and balding of vertex.

c. Type IV male AGA with balding on vertex exceeding 10 cm in diameter.

d. Type IV male AGA with frontal recession of hair.

e. Type V male AGA with intervening bridge of hair between areas of baldness on vertex and frontal area.

f. Type VI male AGA with very little surviving hair between bald areas on vertex and frontal area.

g. Type VII male AGA with total baldness of vertex and frontal area.

Female–Pattern Alopecia

In females the onset of alopecia is significantly delayed over the male counterpart with a similar genetic background, often by a decade. Thus, onset between 25 and 35 years of age is common, and onset at puberty is the exception. The extent of loss in endocrinologically normal females is much more limited than in males. An oval area of thinning is seen over the top of the scalp which may progress through mild to moderate or severe diffuse thinning, with the preservation of an intact frontal hair margin (Figures 3.2a,b,c). This female pattern of diffuse thinning is occasionally seen in men (Figure 3.3). Bitemporal recession of hair may be seen, but usually not of the severity seen in men. If indeed marked bitemporal recession of hair with definite balding of the posterior vertex is seen in women, it is often accompanied by acne and hirsutism, and reflects significant hyperandrogenism (Figure 3.4).

Histopathology

The histopathology of androgenetic alopecia is a reflection of the pathogenesis. Terminal hairs progressively miniaturize and ascend up the follicle to become "vellus" hairs. This change is marked by the presence of residual angiofibrotic tracts which replace the old lower terminal follicle, and are commonly known as streamers or follicular stelae (Figure 3.5a). The net result, seen in horizontal sections of scalp biopsies, is a change in the terminal to "vellus" hair ratio from the normal value of 6:1 or 8:1 to 4:1 or less, and usually of the order of 2:1 in the established case. This is accompanied by an increase in follicular streamers (Figures 3.5b,c). Mild lymphohistocytic inflammation is found around the upper follicle in approximately one-third of normal controls and one-third of cases of androgenetic alopecia, but moderate inflammation is found in another third of cases of androgenetic alopecia (Figure 3.5d) but not in normal controls. The histopathological findings are the same in both male and female androgenetic alopecia with terminal hair depletion and a corresponding increase in "vellus" hairs and stelae, although slightly less "vellus" hairs may be found in the female. There is usually no appreciable reduction in the number of hair follicles although this can occur in 10% of cases.

Investigation and Diagnosis

The diagnosis is usually straightforward when the clinical presentation and family history are considered. Central scalp alopecia of variable pattern and degree is expected. In males bitemporal recession is often prominent. Close inspection of areas of apparent thinning should reveal short hairs scattered throughout the area. These short hairs are the intermediate and "vellus" hairs which represent the progressive miniaturization of terminal hairs as the alopecia proceeds.

Evaluation of common baldness has been facilitated by the use of grading scales developed by Hamilton (1951) and modified by Norwood (1975) *(continued)*

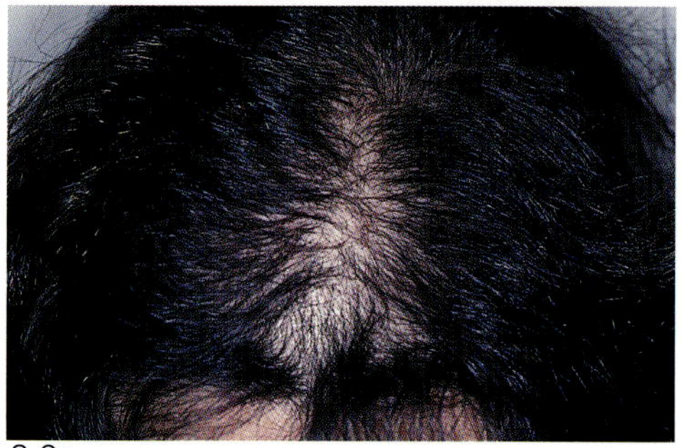

3.2a →

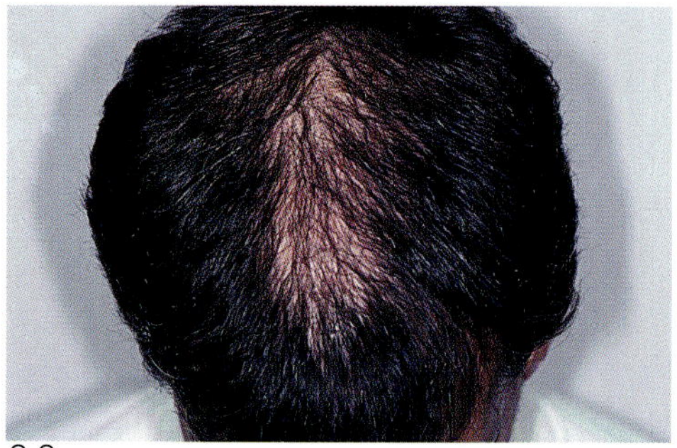

3.3

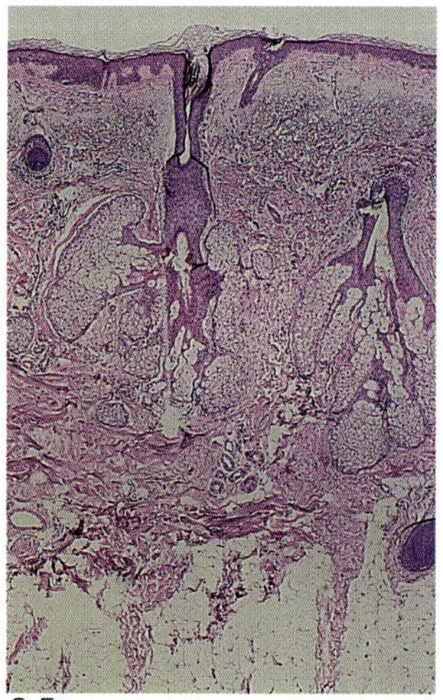

3.5a →

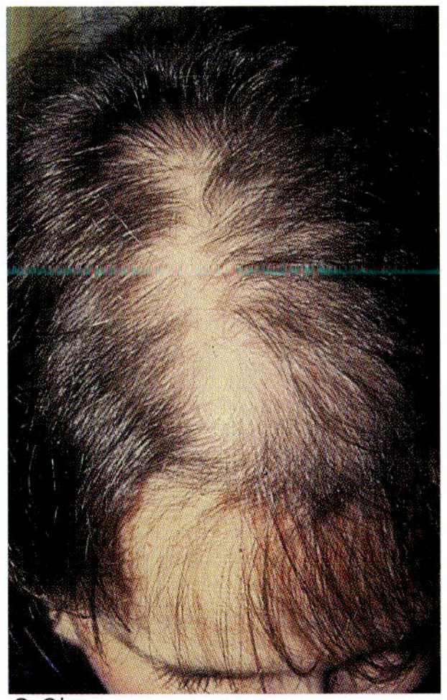

3.2b ➔

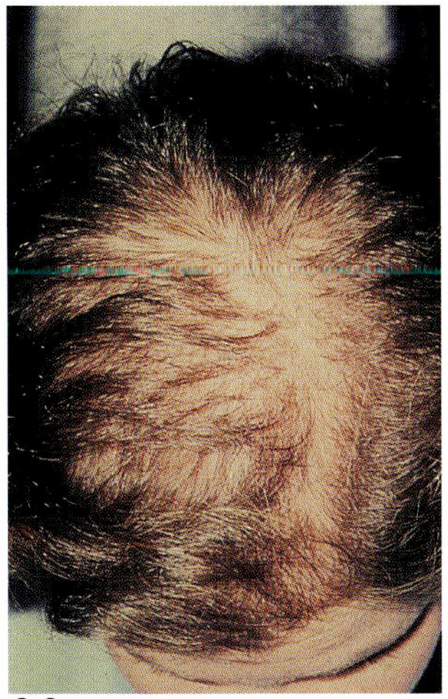

3.2c ■

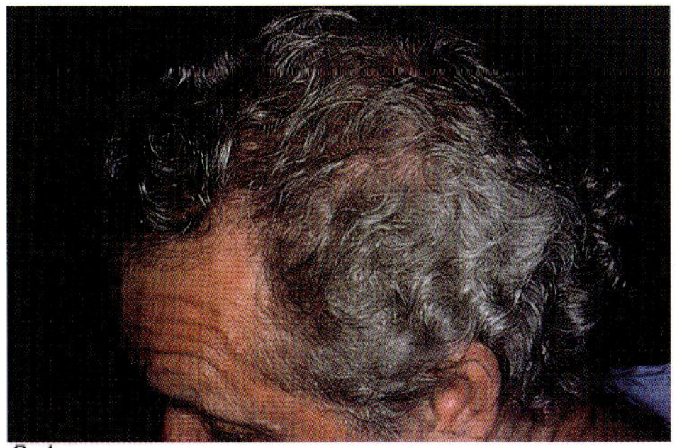

3.4

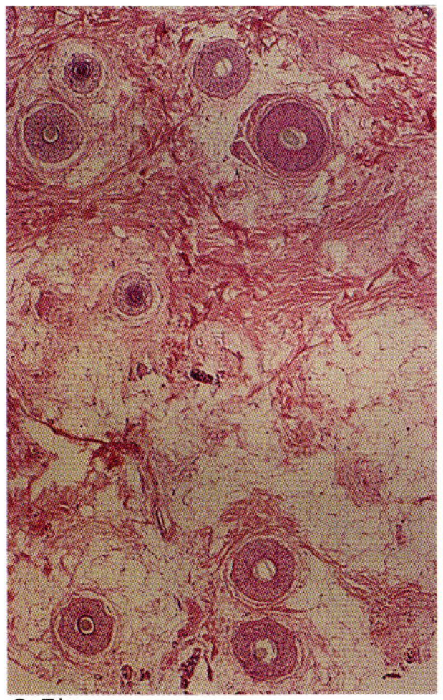

3.5b ➔

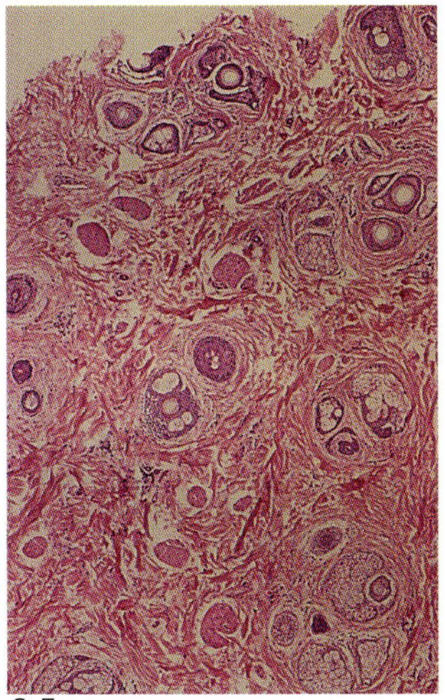

3.5c ➔

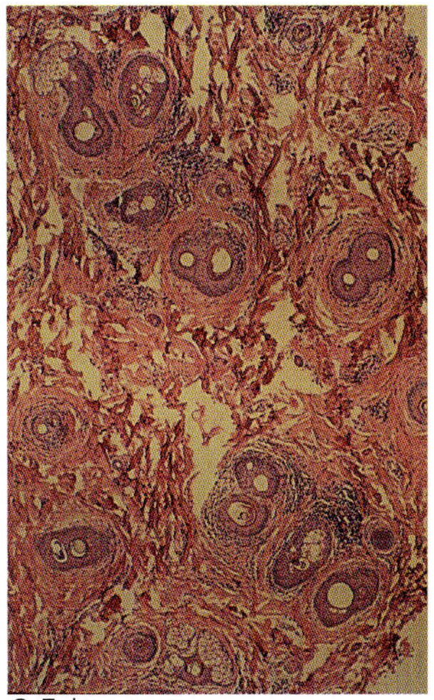

3.5d ■

3.2
Ludwig classification: Female AGA:

a. Mild female AGA with intact frontal hairline and widening of center part.

b. Moderate female AGA with intact frontal hairline and moderate diffuse thinning of hair on top of scalp.

c. Severe female AGA with intact frontal hairline and marked thinning of hair on top of scalp .

3.3
A male with AGA showing female pattern of diffuse thinning over top of scalp with intact frontal hairline.

3.4
AGA in the female with a male pattern of marked bitemporal recession and severe thinning of hair on vertex, due to severe hyperandrogenism.
(*Courtesy of Anne Lucky, M.D.*)

3.5
Scalp biopsy: Histopathology of AGA:

a. Vertical section: The relative lack of terminal hairs projecting into the subcutaneous tissue contrasts with the increase numbers of follicular stela or streamers shown here. LM x 40.

b. Horizontal section: Lower dermis: A decreased number of terminal hairs contrasts wlth a relatlve lncrease ln the number of follicular stelae. LM x 40.

c. Horizontal section: Upper dermis: A decreased number of terminal hairs is accompanied by a relative increase in the number of "vellus" hairs. LM x 40.

d. Horizontal section: Upper dermis: A moderate degree of inflammation with perifollicular lymphohistiocytic infiltration and fibrosis is seen in approximately 1/3 of cases of AGA. LM x 40.

(Figures 3.1a,b,c,d,e,f,g). These scales describe the progression from the normal prepubertal scalp (Type I) to the most extensive loss (Type VII). While women exhibit early male–pattern types, they are more likely to have a diffuse form of loss (Figures 3.2a,b,c). The need to accurately define the extent of hair loss and to evaluate the effectiveness of treatment of androgenetic hair loss has resulted in the development of tools to directly compare the density of patient hair to a standard. To this end the Savin Midvertex Density Scales have been developed for clinical use in males and females (Figures 2.7a,b,c,d,e,f,g,h). The use of such scales allows the clinician to evaluate the progression of hair growth and response to therapy more accurately and will become more important as more modes of therapy become available. However, for reliable experimental accuracy, serial hair counts in a freshly clipped target area are still required.

Differential Diagnosis

In males the diagnosis of well established androgenetic alopecia is generally a relatively simple matter, particularly in the presence of a strong family history of common baldness. In younger men the history of relatively abrupt increases in shedding in the absence of objective evidence of pattern loss can be confusing. In such cases other causes of diffuse alopecia, or even a diffuse form of alopecia areata, must be considered.

In women the diagnosis is often more difficult as more diffuse central thinning is common. In women with frontovertical thinning the co-existence of acne and hirsutism should be noted and, if present, endocrinological assessment may be necessary. It may require repeated evaluation over time to conclude that androgenetic alopecia is operative and not one or another form of diffuse alopecia. When the diagnosis is in doubt in either males or females, scalp biopsy may be helpful.

Treatment

The four basic options in the treatment of androgenetic alopecia are to do nothing, or as significant deterioration occurs, to provide medical treatment, surgical treatment, or a hairpiece.

At the present time, the only medical treatment approved by the Food and Drug Administration in the USA is topical minoxidil 2%. This often must be applied twice daily for at least a year for appreciable effects to be observed. Approximately one third of patients will experience visible hair regrowth, usually to a mild degree, and a similar number will develop a downy regrowth; however, some 80% of patients can expect a cessation of hair loss. If the topical minoxidil is helpful, it must be continued indefinitely. Side effects are minimal.

Drugs with antiandrogenic activity which can be used in female androgenetic alopecia include spironolactone, and cyproterone, which is not available in the USA. The search for an antiandrogen which can safely be used in males continues. In a recent 12-month pilot study of some 200 male patients with androgenetic alopecia, oral finasteride 5mg. daily, as an investigative drug in the treatment of male androgenetic alopecia, was compared with placebo. Preliminary analysis of data showed significantly more hair regrowth in the finasteride than in the placebo patients, and no serious adverse effects were encountered. Dosage studies indicated that 0.2mg. finasteride reduced dihydrotestosterone levels in the scalp as effectively as 5mg. finasteride. Further clinical dose ranging studies of finasteride in male androgenetic alopecia were initiated.

Lack of response to medical treatment or an advanced degree of alopecia may indicate a surgical approach. The advent of minigrafts and micrografts has led to greatly improved cosmetic results. Scalp reductions and the rotation of flaps are also appropriate in selected cases. Complete or partial hairpieces are available, and in males at least need to be custom–fitted. Hair weaves in general are discouraged since they can cause traction alopecia. ■

Suggested Reading

Abell, E.: "Pathology of male pattern alopecia" (abstract). *Arch Dermatol* 1984;120:1607.

Adachi, K., Takayasu, S., Takushima, I., et al.: "Human hair follicles: metabolism and control mechanisms." *J Soc Cosmet Chem* 1970;21:901.

Bergfeld, W.F.: "Skin biopsy findings in androgenic alopecia." *Cutis* 1978;22:195.

Bergfeld, W.F., Redmond, G.P.: "Androgenic alopecia." *Dermatol Clin* 1987;5:491– 500.

Cash, T.F.: "The psychological effects of androgenetic alopecia in men." *J Am Acad Dermatol* 1992;26:926–931

Dawber, R.P.R.: "Special symposium on dermatological therapy." *V. Disease of the appendages, alopecia, and hirsutism. Clin Exp Dermatol* 1982;7:177–182.

DeVillez, R.L.: "Androgenetic alopecia treated with topical minoxidil." *J Am Acad Dermatol* 1987;16:669–672.

DeVillez, R.L.: "Topical minoxidil therapy in hereditary androgenetic alopecia." *Arch Dermatol* 1985;121:197–202.

DeVillez, R.L., Dunn, J.: "The 3 alpha, 17 beta-androstanediol glucuronide/sex hormone binding globulin ratio as a possible marker for female pattern baldness." *Arch Dermatol* 1986;122:1011–1015.

Hamilton, J.B.: "Patterned loss of hair in man: Types and incidence." *Annals of the New York Academy of Sciences* 1951;53:708–728.

Jenkins, E.P., Andersson, S., Imperato-McGinley, J., et al.: "Genetic and pharmacological evidence for more than one human steroid 5 alpha-reductase." *J Clin Invest* 1992;89:293–300.

Kasick, J.M., Bergfeld, W.F., Steck, W.D., et al.: "Adrenal androgenic female- pattern alopecia: sex hormones and the balding woman." *Cleve Clin Q* 1983;50:111–122.

Katz, H.I., Hien, N.T., Prawer, S.E., et al.: "Long-term efficacy of topical minoxidil in male pattern baldness." *J Am Acad Dermatol* 1987;16:711–718.

Kaufman, K.D., DeVillez, R., Roberts, J., et al: "A 12 month pilot clinical study of the effects of finasteride on men with male pattern baldness." *Poster: Abstract Number 550. SID, 55th Annual Meeting.* Baltimore, 4-27-94.

Kuster, W., Happle, R.: "The inheritance of common baldness: two B or not two B?" *J Am Acad Dermatol* 1984;11:921–926.

Ludwig, E.: "Classification of the types of androgenetic alopecia (common baldness), arising in the female sex." *Br J Dermatol* 1977;97:247–254.

Miller, J.A., Darby, C.R., Karkavitsas, K., et al.: "Low sex hormone binding globulin levels in young women with diffuse hair loss." *Br J Dermatol* 1982;106:331–336.

Norwood, O.T.: "Male pattern baldness: classification and incidence." In: Norwood, O.T., (Ed.): *Hair Transplant Surgery.* Springfield: Charles C. Thomas, 1973:3–16.

Olsen, E.A., DeLong, E.R., Weiner, M.S.: "Long-term follow-up of men with male pattern baldness treated with topical minoxidil." *J Am Acad Dermatol* 1987;16:688– 695.

Olsen, E.A.: "Androgenetic alopecia." In: *Disorders of Hair Growth. Diagnosis and Treatment,* Olsen, E.A. (Ed.). New York: McGraw-Hill 1994, 257–283.

Price, V.: "Androgenetic Alopecia." In: Theirs, B.H., Dobson, R.L., Eds. *Pathogenesis of Skin Disease.* New York: Churchill Livingstone, 1986:41–55.

Price, V.H.: "Testosterone metabolism in the skin." *Arch Dermatol* 1975;111:1496– 1502.

Randall, V.A., Thornton, M.J., Hamada, K., et al.: "Mechanism of androgen action in cultured dermal papilla cells derived from human hair follicles with varying responses to androgen in vivo." *J Invest Dermatol* 1992;98:86S–91S.

Reitschel, R.L., Duncan, S.H.: "Safety and efficacy of topical minoxidil in the management of androgenetic alopecia." *J Am Acad Dermatol* 1987;16:677–686.

Savin, R.C.: "Use of topical minoxidil in the treatment of male pattern baldness." *J Am Acad Dermatol* 1987;16:696–704.

Savin, R.C.: "A method for visually describing hair loss in both male and female androgen alopecia." *Poster Exhibit #23, 24. 51st Annual Meeting, American Academy of Dermatology.* San Francisco, 1992.

Sawaya, M.E.: "Purification of androgen receptors in human sebocytes and hair." *J Invest Dermatol* 1992;98:92S–96S.

Shupack, J.L., Kassimir, J.J., Thirumoorthy, T., et al.: "Dose response study of topical minoxidil in male pattern alopecia." *J Am Acad Dermatol* 1987;16:673–676.

Trueb, R.M.: "Female pattern baldness in men." *J Am Acad Dermatol* 1993;29:782– 783.

Whiting, D.A.: "Diagnostic and predictive value of horizontal sections of scalp biopsy specimens in male pattern androgenetic alopecia." *J Am Acad Dermatol* 1993;28:755–763.

Diffuse Alopecia

Definition

Diffuse alopecia is defined here as a generalized, or global, thinning of hair over the entire scalp. It is often inconspicuous since severe hair loss is necessary before diffuse alopecia becomes visible. The course of diffuse global alopecia is variable and can be continuous or episodic, depending on the cause.

Etiology

The many causes of diffuse alopecia can be grouped under the headings shown in Table 4.1.

Clinical Description

Telogen Effluvium:
Telogen effluvium is a diffuse loss of normal club hairs from normal resting follicles. It is usually due to a premature interruption of growth in many anagen hairs which then cycle through catagen into a telogen phase, so that the proportion of telogen hairs rises above the normal 5-10%. When the resting phase ends 2-4 months later, new anagen hairs displace the club hairs which loosen and fall out abruptly in large numbers, often enough to block the drain in the shower (Figures 4.1a,b,c). Causes include childbirth (Figure 4.2), febrile illnesses, surgical operations, chronic systemic disease, crash diets (Figure 4.3), traction, severe emotional stress, physiological alopecia in the newborn, and many different drugs including antithyroid drugs, anticoagulants, beta blockers, sodium valproate and others (Table 4.2). In the acute phase, hair pull tests are positive all over the scalp, yielding abnormally high numbers of telogen hairs. Significant bitemporal recession of hair is often a prominent feature of telogen effluvium, often exceeding the recession seen in female androgenetic alopecia, where preservation of an intact and often accentuated frontal hairline is the rule. This recession is of much less significance in males, in whom telogen effluvium is infrequent. The diffuse thinning is only visible if the hair loss is severe. Telogen effluvium usually remits within 3-6 months, when caused by a single episode such as childbirth, a febrile illness or a crash diet (Figures 4.4a,b,c,d). However, some cases of telogen effluvium persist for much longer periods. This is particularly true when the cause is not removed, or if other mechanisms such as telogen arrest, short anagen cycles, or idiopathic causes, are involved. (See Idiopathic Diffuse Alopecia including Chronic Telogen Effluvium.)

(continued)

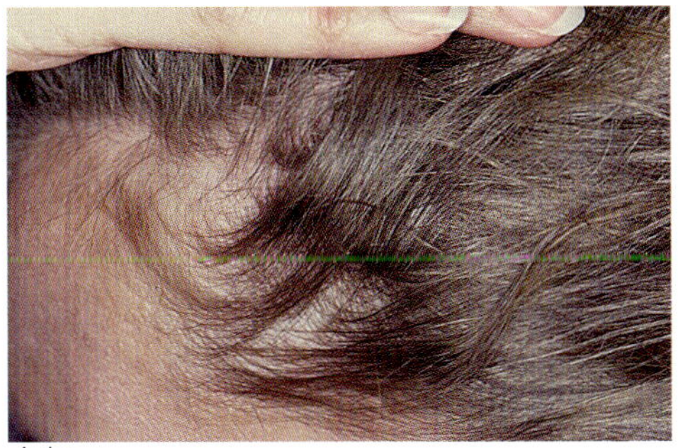

4.1a →

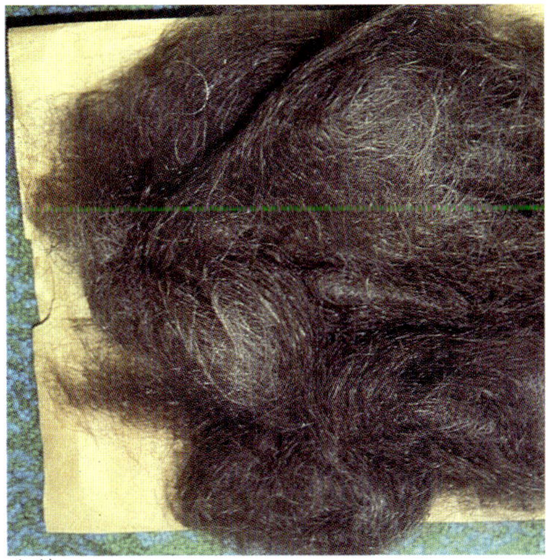

4.1b →

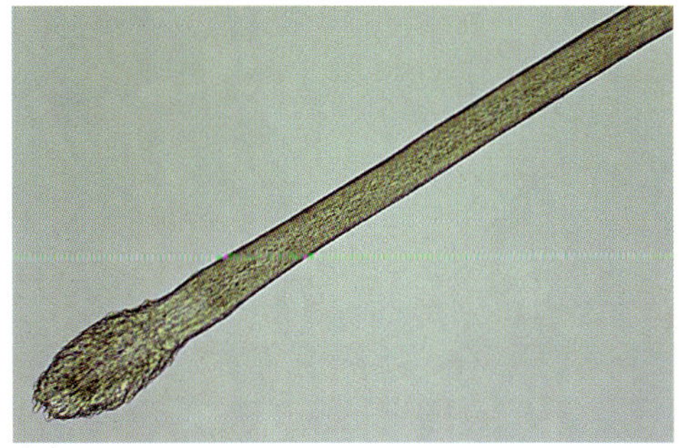

4.1c ■

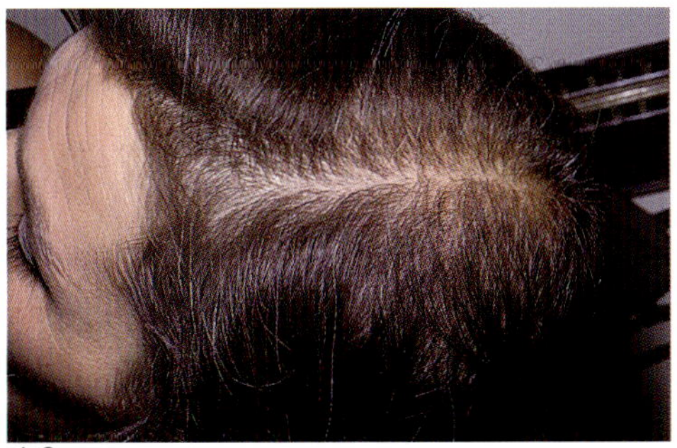

4.2

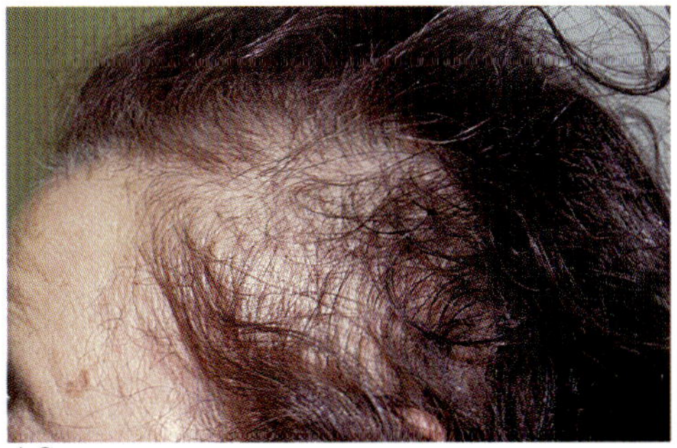

4.3

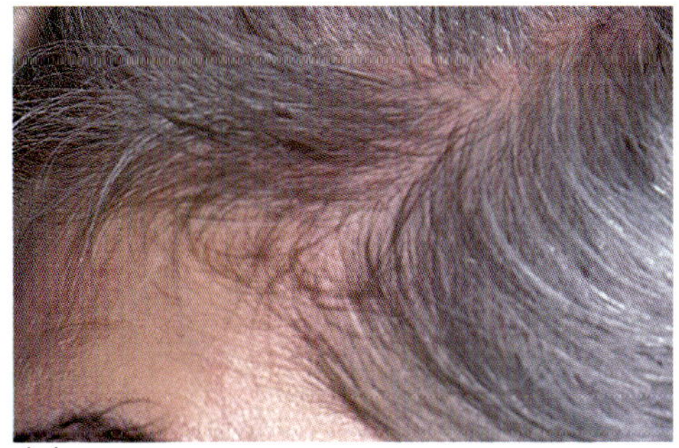

4.4a →

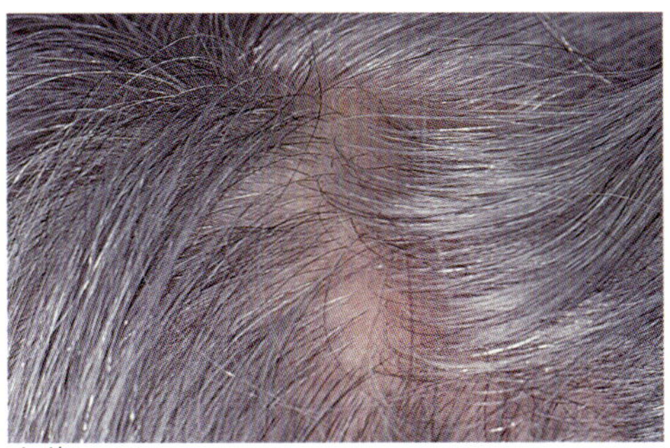

4.4b →

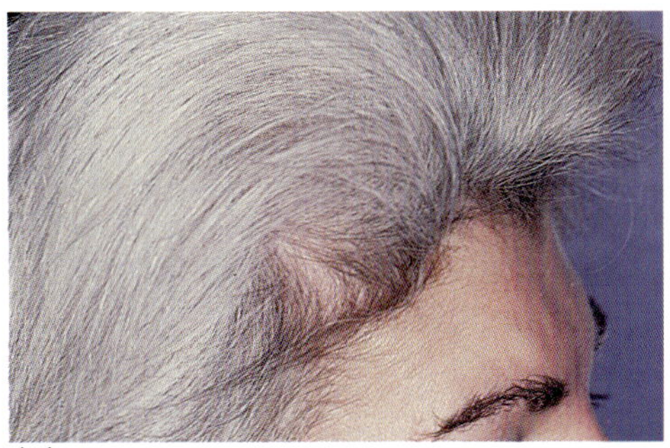

4.4c →

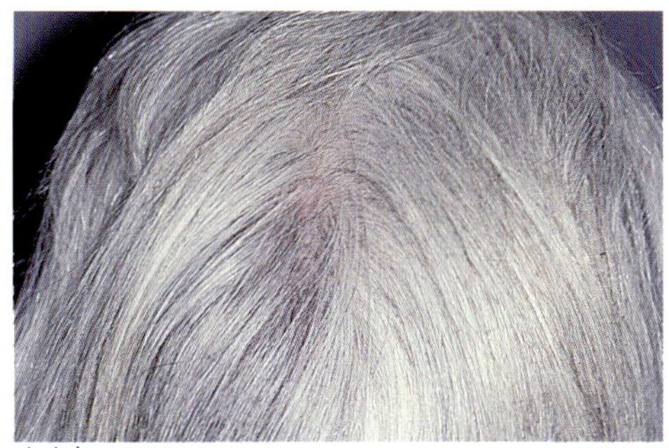

4.4d ■

4.1
Diffuse alopecia: Telogen effluvium:

a. Obvious temporal recession with diffuse alopecia of abrupt onset is characteristic of telogen effluvium.

b. The patient often produces handfuls of hair as evidence of the severe hair loss.

c. Club hair: The hairs extracted from the patient's head by a pull test, or the patient's shed hairs, all prove to be club or telogen hairs. These hairs lack a root sheath, have an expanded bulb, and lack pigment in and around the bulb. LM x 100. *(Reprinted with permission, Whiting, D.A., The Diagnosis of Alopecia, Current Concepts, Upjohn, 1990.)*

4.2
Diffuse alopecia: Telogen effluvium, post-partum: Diffuse thinning of hair all over scalp with recession in temples.

4.3
Diffuse alopecia: Telogen effluvium due to crash diet: Marked temporal recession of hair is seen with diffuse hair loss.

4.4
Diffuse alopecia: Telogen effluvium, hair loss and regrowth:

a. Marked temporal thinning of hair.

b. The widespread thinning of hair is seen here over the occipital area.

c. Marked regrowth of hair in temples 4 months later.

d. The general regrowth of hair is seen here over the occipital area, 4 months later.

Table 4.1 Causes of diffuse alopecia*

Telogen effluvium	Nutritional
Anagen effluvium	Malabsorption
Drugs	Renal failure
Other chemicals	Hepatic failure
Thyroid disorders	Systemic disease
Iron deficiency	Miscellaneous
Hereditary and congenital	Idiopathic diffuse global alopecia including chronic telogen effluvium

*After Rook, A., Dawber, R.: Diseases of the Hair and Scalp (2nd Ed). Oxford: Blackwell Scientific Publications, 1991:136–166.

Table 4.2 Drugs which may cause telogen effluvium*

Amphetamine
Angiotensin converting enzyme inhibitors: Captopril, Enalapril
Anticoagulants: Dextran sulfate, Dicumarol, Heparin, Warfarin
Anticonvulsants: Carbamazepine, Ethotoin, Mephenytoin, Paramethadione, Phenytoin Trimethadione, Valproate sodium
Antithyroid drugs: Carbimazole, Iodine, Methimazole, Methylthiouracil, Propylthiouracil
Beta Blockers: Acebutolol, Atenolol, Labetalol, Metoprolol, Nadolol, Pindolol, Propranolol, Timolol
Birth Control Drugs
Bromocriptine
Calcium Channel Blockers: Verapamil
Cholesterol Reducers: Cholestyramine, Clofibrate, Nicotinic acid, Triparanol
Cimetidine
Danazol
Levodopa
Lithium
Methysergide
Metyrapone
Nitrofurantoin
Nonsteroidal Anti–inflammatories: Ibuprofen
Pyridostigmine Bromide
Retinoids and Retinol: Acitretin, Etretinate, Isotretinoin, Vitamin A overdose
Salicylates: Aminosalicylic acid

*After Headington, J.T.: Telogen effluvium: New concepts and review. Arch Dermatol 1993;129:356–363.

Anagen Effluvium:
Anagen effluvium is characterized by the diffuse loss of anagen hairs from growing follicles. Arrested cell division in the hair-bulb matrix leads to progressive narrowing of the hair shaft or to failure of hair formation. The weakened hairs easily fracture and their proximal ends are tapered (pencil pointing). Anagen alopecia occurs within a few weeks, and if the inhibitory influence is removed, hairs will regrow promptly in anagen follicles. Causes of anagen effluvium include cytostatic drugs, x-ray therapy, endocrine diseases, alopecia areata, cicatricial alopecia, trauma and pressure, severe protein calorie malnutrition, such as kwashiorkor and marasmus, and other toxic drugs such as arsenic, bismuth, borax, colchicine, gold and thallium (Table 4.3). The diffuse alopecia is severe and clinically obvious, since anagen hairs are affected and they represent the majority of the hairs on the scalp (Figure 4.5a). The affected hair shafts may show one or more constrictions, depending on the degree of continuous or intermittent inhibition of mitosis. Hairs are readily detached by pull tests and many will show proximal, tapered fractures (Figure 4.5b). Pluck tests may be misleading in advanced cases of anagen effluvium because telogen hairs may be all that remain in the scalp.

(continued)

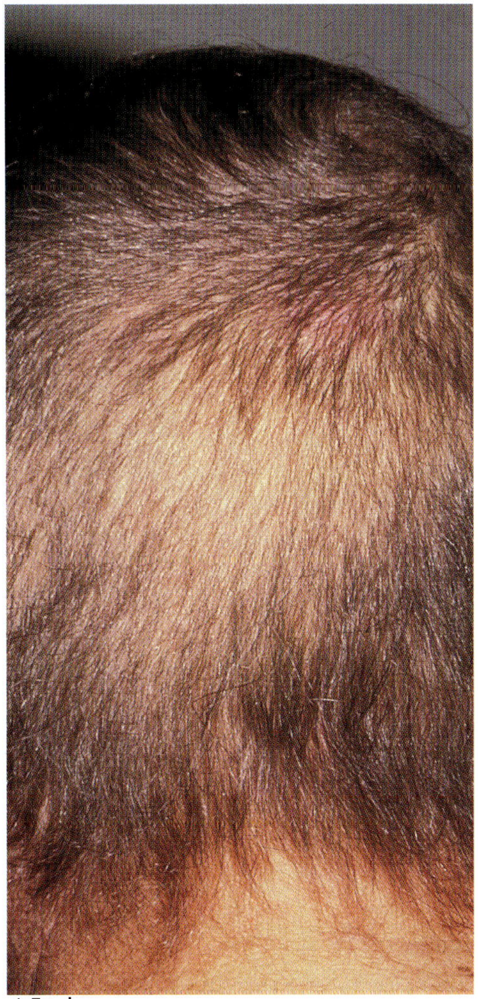

4.5a ↓

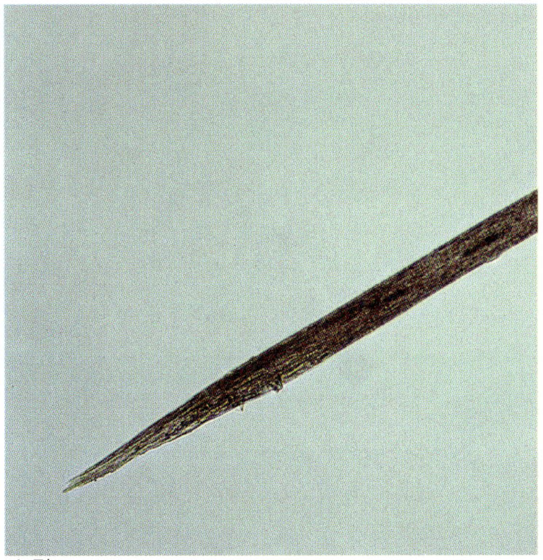

4.5b ■

4.5
Diffuse alopecia: Anagen effluvium:

a. Marked thinning of hair all over the scalp. *(Reprinted with permission, Whiting, D.A., J. Am. Acad. Dermatol., 1987.)*

b. Broken off hair shows tapering of the proximal end. LM x 40. *(Reprinted with permission, Whiting, D.A., The Diagnosis of Alopecia, Current Concepts, Upjohn, 1990.)*

Table 4.3 Drugs which may cause anagen effluvium

Anticancer drugs:	Bleomycin	Fluorouracil
	Cyclophosphamide	Methotrexate
	Cytarabine	Mitomycin
	Dactinomycin	Mitoxantrone
	Daunorubicin	Procarbazine
	Doxorubicin	Thioguanine
	Etoposide	Vinblastine
	Floxuridine	Vincristine
Miscellaneous drugs:	Arsenic	Colchicine
	Bismuth	Gold
	Borax	Thallium

Drugs and Chemicals:

Alopecia caused by drugs and chemicals is usually confined to the scalp but may also affect facial and body hair. The alopecia is usually diffuse since it is caused by a systemic influence. Drug-related alopecia may present as a telogen or anagen effluvium or may be of a nonspecific dystrophic variety. The mode of action of the drug is frequently unknown and a careful history of all drugs taken in the recent past is important for diagnostic purposes. The best way to confirm the diagnosis of drug–related alopecia is to stop the drug, wait for the hair growth to improve and later rechallenge with the same drug to see if alopecia recurs. Unfortunately, this is not always possible. Alopecia due to drugs is usually reversible except for some cases of cicatricial alopecia due to a lichenoid drug eruption. The list of drugs reported to cause alopecia is constantly increasing. Table 2.3 lists many drugs currently recognized to sometimes be responsible for alopecia.

There are various categories of drugs that can cause alopecia and these are listed in Table 4.4.

There are miscellaneous chemicals that cause alopecia and these are listed in Table 4.5.

Thyroid Disorder:

The alopecia seen in thyroid disorder is of gradual onset and is diffuse with a marked increase in telogen hairs. It may be accompanied by thinning of the outer third of the eyebrows, dry skin, hoarseness, myxedema, weight gain, cold intolerance, and lack of energy and initiative. Thyroid function tests must be done when hypothyroidism is suspected. Hypopituitarism can cause a similar type of hair loss. Cases of alopecia have been described in hyperthyroidism but are difficult to confirm. Alopecia due to thyroid disorder should be reversible when the patient is returned to the euthyroid state.

Iron Deficiency:

Iron deficiency is regarded by many as a cause for alopecia. Some cases of diffuse alopecia may be caused by iron deficiency, but in others the coexistence of diffuse alopecia and iron deficiency may be fortuitous. However, in all cases of diffuse alopecia, a complete blood count and determination of serum iron and ferritin levels are indicated. If iron deficiency is found, the cause should be investigated and treated.

Hereditary and Congenital Diffuse Alopecia:

Diffuse alopecia can occur in a number of inherited and congenital conditions. It may occur as an isolated defect or as part of a syndrome. More details are given in chapter 11.

Table 4.4 Categories of drugs that can cause alopecia

Alpha Receptor Blockers	Doxazosin Terazosin	Prazosin
Angiotensin converting enzyme inhibitors	Captopril	Enalapril
Anticancer drugs	Bleomycin Cyclophosphamide Cytarabine Dactinomycin Daunorubicin Doxorubicin Etoposide Floxuridine	Fluorouracil Methotrexate Mitomycin Mitoxantrone Procarbazine Thioguanine Vinblastine Vincristine
Anticoagulant drugs	Dicumarol Heparin	Warfarin
Anticonvulsant drugs	Ethotoin Mephenytoin Paramethadione	Phenytoin Trimethadione Valproate sodium
Antithyroid drugs	Carbimazole Methimazole	Methylthiouracil Propylthiouracil
Beta Blockers	Acebutolol Atenolol Labetalol Metoprolol	Nadolol Pindolol Propranolol Timolol
Calcium Channel Blockers	Diltiazem	Verapamil
Cholesterol Reducers	Clofibrate	Lovastatin
Histamine H2 receptor blockers	Cimetidine Famotidine	Ranitidine
Nonsteroidal anti–inflammatory drugs	Fenoprofen Ibuprofen Indomethacin Ketoprofen	Meclomen Naproxen Piroxicam Sulindac
Retinoids and retinol	Acitretin Etretinate	Isotretinoin Vitamin A overdose
Tricyclic antidepressants	Amitriptyline Amoxapine Desipramine Doxepin	Imipramine Nortriptyline Protriptyline Trimipramine

Table 4.5 Miscellaneous chemicals that can cause alopecia*

Chemical	Source
Abrin	Plant source, Abrus precatorius
Arsenic	Pesticides
Bismuth	Old treatment for syphilis
Boric acid	Mouth washes, occupational
Chloroprene dimers	Synthetic rubber manufacture
Lead	Paints
Mercury	Cosmetics, teething powders, antispetics
Mimosine	Plant source, Leucaena glauca
Selenocystothione	Plant source, Lecythis
Thallium salts	Rodent poison

*After Rook, A., Dawber, R.: Diseases of the Hair and Scalp (2nd Ed). Oxford: Blackwell Scientific Publications, 1991:136–166.

Nutritional Influences on Hair Growth:
Nutritional influences must be severe to have a significant impact on hair growth. Protein–calorie malnutrition of the magnitude seen in marasmus or kwashiorkor can cause prompt hair loss, presumably from anagen effluvium. Anagen hair roots become dystrophic, with reduction in diameter of root and bulb, the rate of hair growth decreases, and the proportion of telogen hairs increases. In chronic kwashiorkor, hairs may become lusterless and lighter or reddish in color or show intermittent bands of color change, the so called "flag sign." The diffuse alopecia seen with crash diets is usually delayed for 6-10 weeks and corresponds to a telogen effluvium.

Zinc deficiency can cause alopecia, with hairs becoming sparse, fine, and light in color. There is an associated dermatitis of mouth, anus, and extremities. Causes include low zinc levels in maternal breast milk, acrodermatitis enteropathica, and parenteral hyperalimentation.

Essential fatty acid deficiency which can occur in infancy, and in adults receiving prolonged parenteral alimentation, results in red, scaly scalp and eyebrows, and in alopecia with dry, light hair. Children with biotin-responsive multiple carboxylase deficiency and adults receiving long-term, total parenteral nutrition may develop biotin deficiency. Ocular, neurologic, and cutaneous disorders can result, including a scaly erythema and diffuse loss of scalp and body hair.

Malabsorption:
Severe malabsorption which can be seen in tropical sprue, celiac disease, and pancreatic disease, can result in sparse hair and steatorrhea, dry, scaly skin, weight loss, and growth retardation.

Renal Failure:
Diffuse alopecia, brittle nails and hyperpigmentation and dry, itchy skin may result from chronic renal failure due to any cause. Maintenance hemodialysis does not reverse these changes.

Hepatic Failure:
Common features of liver failure are pruritus, prurigo, jaundice, and spider angiomata, but sometimes liver failure can be associated with diffuse alopecia without any other specific features.

(continued)

Systemic Disease:
Severe, febrile illnesses and other acute illnesses can produce delayed alopecia of the telogen effluvium type. Other diseases can be associated with diffuse alopecia. These include secondary syphilis which can produce a "moth–eaten" and patchy appearance (Figure 4.6). Collagen vascular diseases, such as systemic or subacute lupus erythematosus, dermatomyositis, and scleroderma are frequently associated with diffuse alopecia. Advanced metastatic carcinomatosis can also be associated with alopecia.

Miscellaneous:
Miscellaneous causes of diffuse alopecia include the Cronkite–Canada syndrome, in which diarrhea, weakness, and weight loss usually precede diffuse hair loss and nail dystrophy. Various organic lesions of the central nervous system can cause alopecia as can various other diseases.

Idiopathic Diffuse Alopecia including Chronic Telogen Effluvium:
So–called idiopathic diffuse global alopecia occurs in women in whom no obvious cause can be found and in whom no family history of alopecia can be elicited. Overlapping female androgenetic alopecia and alopecia areata may be recognized in some cases. However, there is a significant group of middle–aged women, often with dense hair, who experience an abrupt diffuse hair loss all over the scalp. This is similar to that seen with telogen effluvium but appears to be much more chronic in that it can persist for years. It is often characterized by bitemporal recession of hair which tends to advance and recede. Episodic shedding occurs which may be seasonal. Specific etiologic factors are difficult to identify. There appears to be a problem of hair cycling in these patients resulting in an increased proportion of hairs in telogen on an intermittent basis. The hair loss in these patients causes extreme anxiety, but nonetheless, the patients do not go bald despite the extensive effluvium. The likely diagnosis in these patients is that of chronic telogen effluvium of unknown etiology.

Histopathology of Chronic Telogen Effluvium

The histopathology of diffuse alopecia is not striking, and in vertical sections of scalp biopsies does not differ from that seen in biopsies of normal scalp (Figure 4.7a). There is no increase in follicular stelae or streamers such as seen in androgenetic alopecia. With horizontal sections of scalp biopsies, follicular counts show that the total number of hairs is normal and the terminal to "vellus" hair ratio is normal at approximately nine terminal hairs to one "vellus" hair (Figures 4.7b,c). The anagen to telogen ratio is very slightly changed in that there are some 89% anagen hairs to 11% telogen hairs. The usual finding is that there is neither absence of hair follicles, nor miniaturization of follicles.

Investigation and Diagnosis

The diagnosis of diffuse alopecia can usually be made with confidence on clinical grounds. However, it is sometimes difficult to distinguish from diffuse female androgenetic alopecia of the vertex and possibly from an early diffuse severe form of alopecia areata, and scalp biopsies may be necessary. Routine tests should include a complete blood count, routine serum chemistry, urinalysis, a thyroid profile, and serological test for syphilis.

Differential Diagnosis

Diffuse alopecia can sometimes be confused with a diffuse form of androgenetic alopecia and also with an early severe diffuse alopecia areata. If there is a long history of alopecia, then hereditary and congenital forms of diffuse alopecia and hypotrichosis should be excluded.

Treatment

The treatment of diffuse alopecia depends on identifying the cause. Any causative drugs should be identified and, if possible, discontinued. Any underlying disease should be identified and treated appropriately. Cases of acute telogen effluvium due to an isolated event are usually self–limiting and should not require treatment. Cases of chronic telogen effluvium, which may account for many cases of diffuse global alopecia, may benefit from topical minoxidil. ■

4.6
Diffuse alopecia: Secondary syphilis. *(Courtesy of H. Francois Jordaan, M. Med.)*

4.7
Scalp biopsy: Histopathology of chronic telogen effluvium:

a. Vertical section: A normal density of terminal hairs projects into the subcutaneous tissue. Follicular stelae are not present here. LM x 40.

b. Horizontal section: Lower dermis: Large numbers of terminal anagen hairs contrast with relatively few follicular stelae. No inflammatory change. LM x 40.

c. Horizontal section: Upper dermis: Many terminal hairs contrast with few vellus hairs. LM x 40.

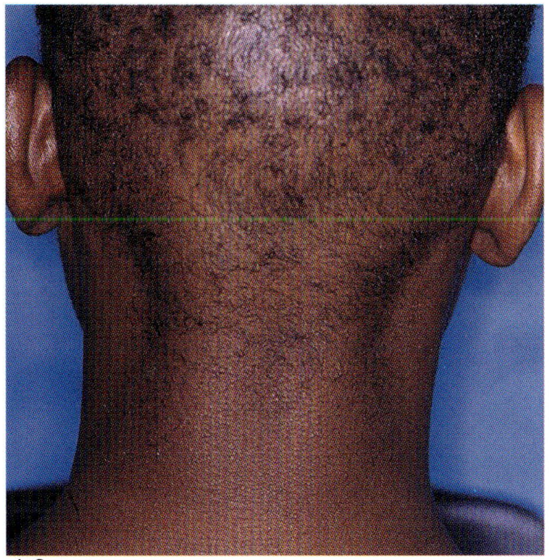

4.6

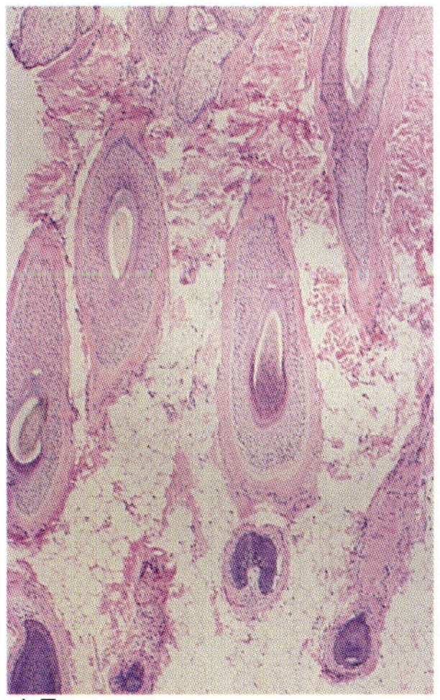

4.7a ↓

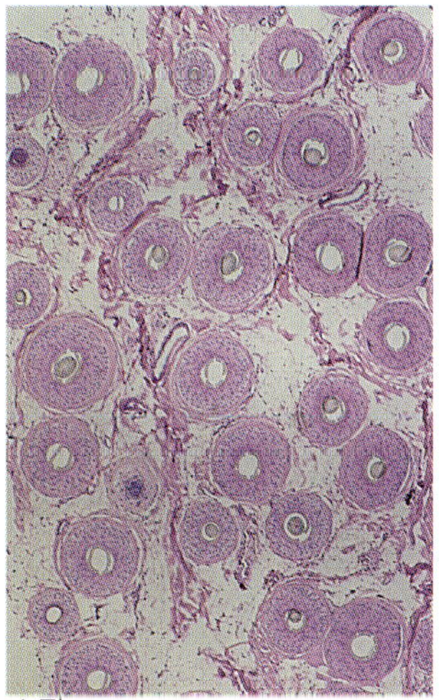

4.7b ↓

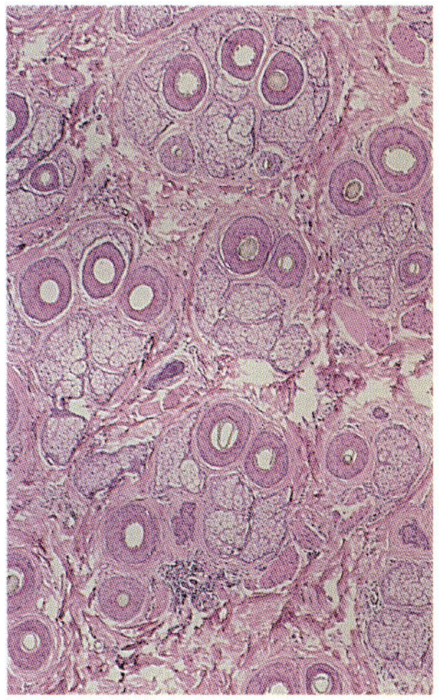

4.7c ■

Suggested Reading

Banks, W.J., Pleasure, D.E., Suzuki, K., et al.: "Thallium poisoning." *Arch Neurol* 1972;26:456–464.

Berth-Jones, J., Shuttleworth, D., Hutchinson, P.E.: "A study of etretinate alopecia." *Br J Dermatol* 1990;122:751–755.

Blankenship, M.L.: "Drugs and alopecia." *Australia J Dermatol* 1983;24:100–104.

Cornbleet, T., Hoit, C.: "Alopecia from coumadin." *Arch Dermatol Syphilol* 1957;75:440–441.

Crounse, R.G., Van Scott, E.J.: "Changes in scalp hair roots as a measure of toxicity from cancer chemotherapeutic drugs." *J Invest Dermatol* 1960;35:83–90.

Fiedler, V.C., Hafeez, A.: "Diffuse alopecia: Telogen hair loss." In: *Disorders of Hair Growth. Diagnosis and Treatment,* Olsen, E.A. (Ed.). New York: McGraw-Hill 1994, 241–255

Freinkel, R.K., Freinkel, N.: "Hair growth and alopecia in hypothyroidism." *Arch Dermatol* 1972;106:349–352.

Grossman, K.L., Kvedar, J.C.: "Anagen hair loss." In: *Disorders of Hair Growth. Diagnosis and Treatment,* Olsen, E.A. (Ed.). New York: McGraw-Hill 1994, 223–239.

Gummer, C.L.: "Diet and hair loss." *Semin Dermatol* 1985;4:35–39.

Headington, J.T.: "Telogen effluvium: New concepts and review." *Arch Dermatol* 1993;129:356–363.

Holick, M.F.: "Vitamin D resistance and alopecia. A causal or casual relationship." *Arch Dermatol* 1985;121:601–603.

Jillson, O.F.: "Alopecia. IV. Diffuse hair loss (nonscarring)." *Cutis* 1983;31:465,469,472.

Kaufman, J.P.: "Telogen effluvium secondary to starvation diet." *Arch Dermatol* 1976;112:731.

Kligman, A.M.: "Pathologic dynamics of human hair loss I: Telogen effluvium." *Arch Dermatol* 1961;83:175–198.

Lynfield, Y.L.: "Effect of pregnancy on the human hair cycle." *J Invest Dermatol* 1960;35:323–327.

Paus R., Stenn, K.S., Link, R.E.: "Telogen skin contains an inhibitor of hair growth." *Br J Dermatol* 1990;122:777–784.

Rook, A., Dawber, R.: *Diseases of the Hair and Scalp (2nd ed.).* Oxford: Blackwell Scientific Publications, 1991:136–166.

Sperling, L.C.: "Transverse anatomy of telogen effluvium." *J Assoc Milit Dermatol* 1990;16:3–10

Steck, W.D.: "Telogen effluvium: A clinically useful concept, with traction alopecia as an example." *Cutis* 1978;21:543–548.

Stroud, J.D.: "Drug–induced alopecia." *Semin Dermatol* 1985;4:29–34.

Van Scott, E.J., Ekel, T.M., Auerbach, R.: "Determinants of rate and kinetics of cell division in scalp hair." *J Invest Dermatol* 1963;41:269–273.

Williams, M.L., Packman, S., Cowan, M.J.: Alopecia and perioral dermatitis in biotin–responsive multiple carboxylase deficiency." *J Am Acad Dermatol* 1983;9:97–103.

Alopecia Areata

Definition

Alopecia areata is the symptomless loss of hair in small circumscribed patches which may remain discrete or may expand into total loss of all scalp and even body hair. It is further defined by being non-scarring, reversible and without known predilection for age, sex, or race.

Etiology

A number of etiologic factors have been considered; however, the precise etiology remains obscure. The most popular current hypothesis considers alopecia areata to be an organ-specific autoimmune disease. The finding of immunoreactants within the hair follicle in active alopecia areata has been inconsistent, but helper T-cells are consistently found in the lymphocyte-rich infiltrate around the affected hair bulb. Support for the autoimmune hypothesis comes from the association of alopecia areata with other known autoimmune conditions, such as Hashimoto's disease, pernicious anemia, Addison's disease, systemic lupus erythematosus, and vitiligo.

There is evidence of a genetic predisposition to alopecia areata. A family history of alopecia areata is present in some 20% of cases. Several studies have shown alopecia areata in twins. The results of HLA studies have failed to show consistent associations, although recent work in the USA has shown the importance of DR4, DR5 (1101) and DQw3 genes in susceptibility to alopecia areata, and of DRw52a and DQ beta 603 in resistance to alopecia areata. Genetic predisposition may be mediated through genetically determined characteristics of immune function.
The increased association of alopecia areata with both the atopic state and Down's syndrome is well established. The associated increased incidence of anti-thyroid antibodies in Down's syndrome patients with alopecia areata, supports the autoimmune hypothesis above.

Emotional stress has long been considered a precipitating factor in many cases of alopecia areata. Efforts to substantiate such a causative role for stress have resulted in such divergent findings as to be of little benefit. Regardless, most clinicians appear to accept significant emotional stress as an important trigger factor in at least some cases of alopecia areata. Even here, the effect of stress on immunologic function may be the important link.

Clinical Description

The typical patient with alopecia areata notes the sudden appearance of a circular patch of hair loss (Figure 5.1). Areas of activity in the lesion may be indicated by the presence of "exclamation point" hairs (Figure 5.2) which are usually 3-4 mm long and may have a dark expanded tip and a depigmented root (Figure 2.9). This usually asymptomatic lesion is found most commonly in the scalp and is noted as a smooth, totally bald area. Initial areas of loss can of course occur on any hair bearing area. Loss of eyebrows and eyelashes or patches of beard in dark-haired men can be most dramatic and conspicuous. In fair-haired individuals patches outside the scalp may go unnoticed.

The course of alopecia areata is unpredictable. The initial patch may regrow spontaneously within a few months, may remain relatively unchanged, may be joined by additional patches over a period of several weeks (Figure 5.3) or may dramatically proceed to large patches of loss (Figure 5.4) or total baldness. The complete loss of scalp hair is referred to as alopecia totalis (Figure 5.5a) and the complete loss of all scalp and body hair is referred to as alopecia universalis (Figure 5.5b).

(continued)

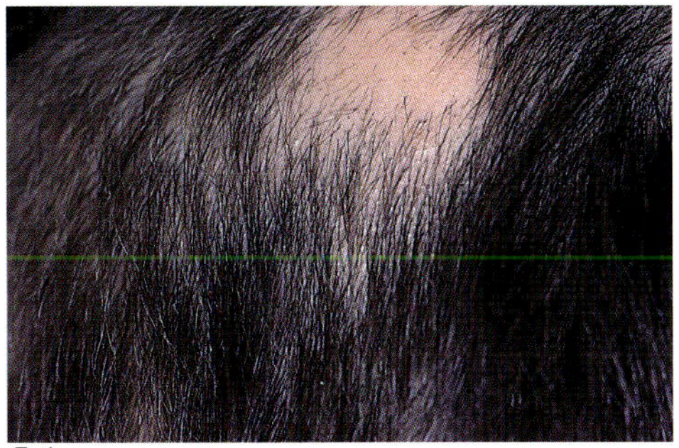
5.1

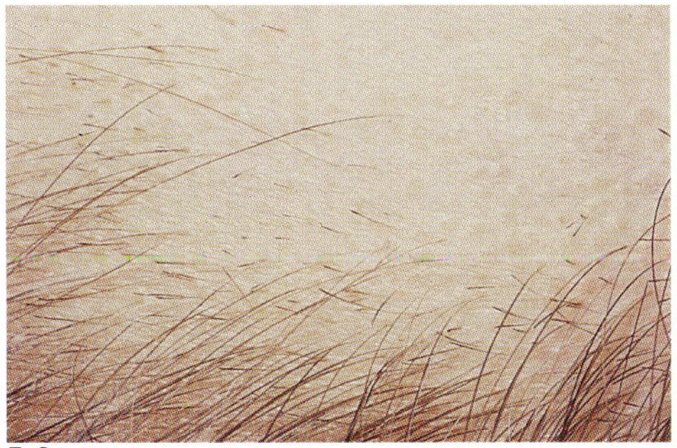
5.2

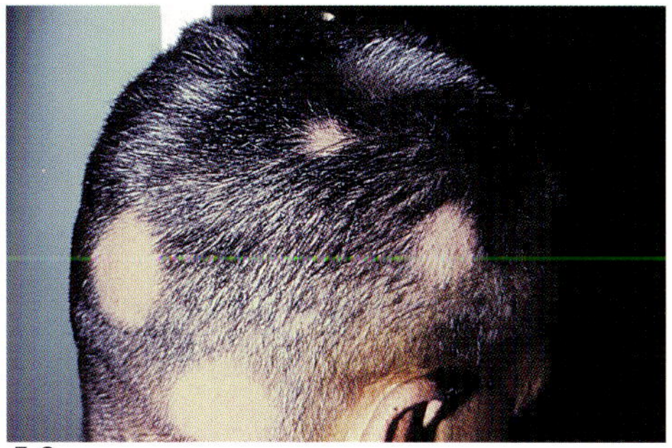
5.3

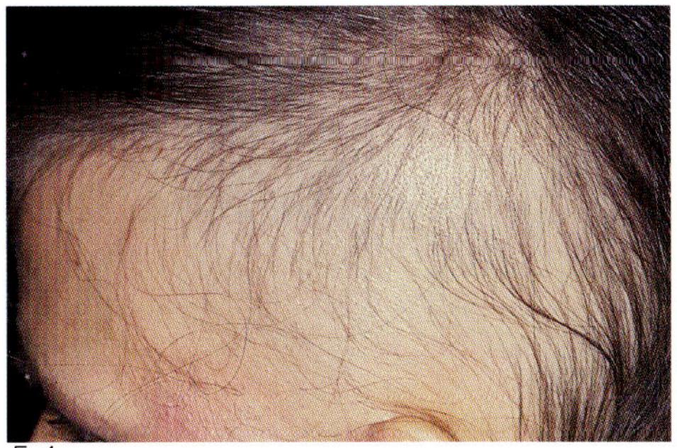
5.4

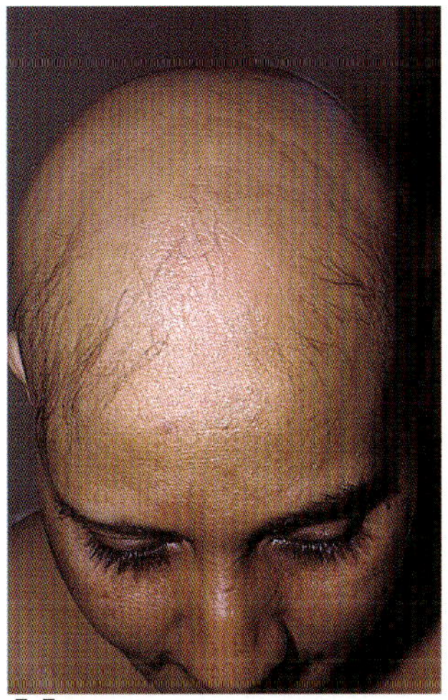
5.5a ➔

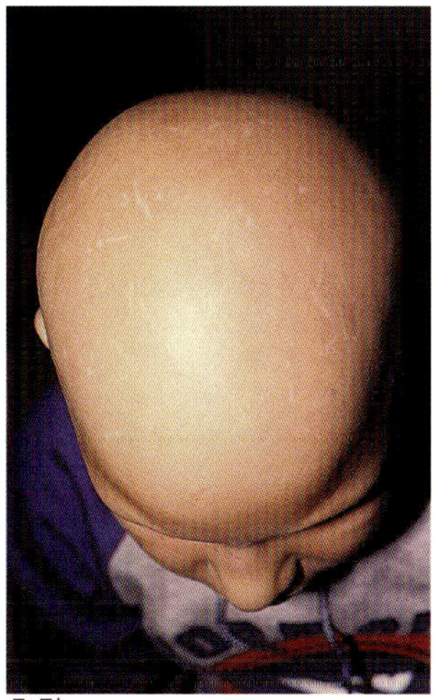
5.5b ■

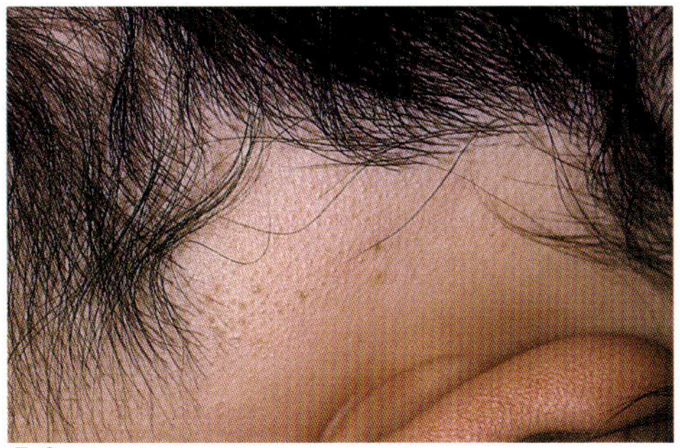
5.6a ➔

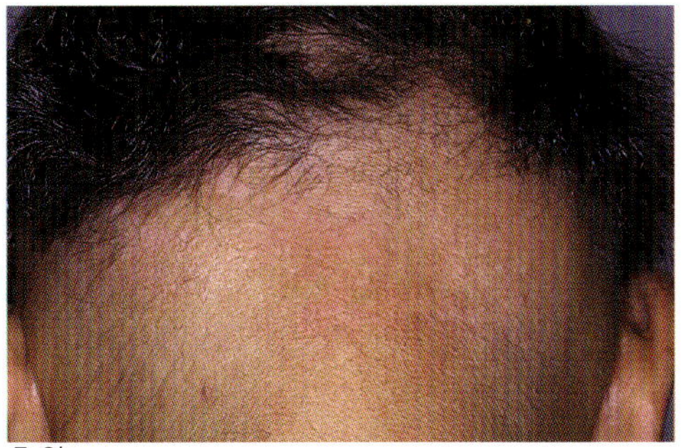
5.6b ■

5.1
Alopecia areata: Single, round patch of alopecia with smooth, peach colored appearance and an active advancing border containing some exclamation point hairs.

5.2
Alopecia areata: Exclamation point hairs at advancing edge of patch of alopecia.

5.3
Alopecia areata: Multiple round patches of alopecia in a young patient.

5.4
Alopecia areata: Diffuse hair loss.

5.5
Alopecia areata:

a. Alopecia totalis: Affects whole scalp but spares eyebrows and eyelashes.

b. Alopecia universalis: Total hair loss from scalp, eyebrows and eyelashes.

5.6
Alopecia areata: Ophiasis.

a. Early ophiasis.

b. Extensive ophiasis.

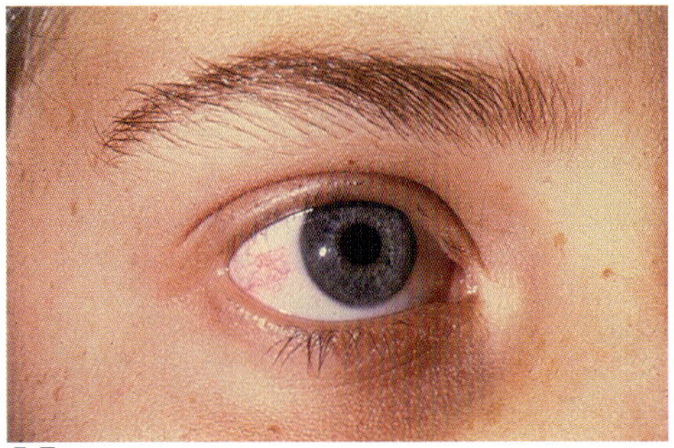
5.7a →

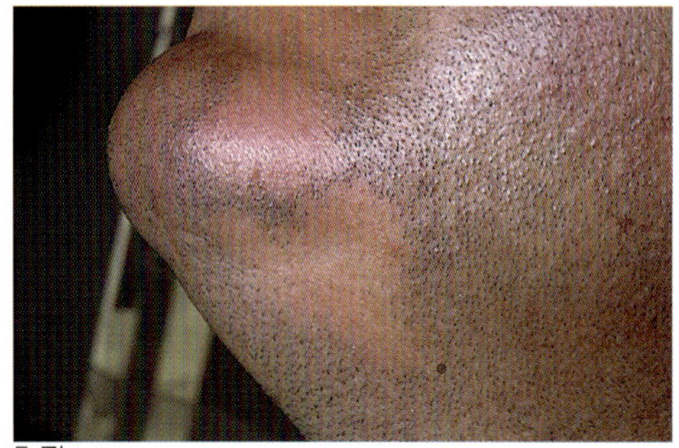
5.7b →

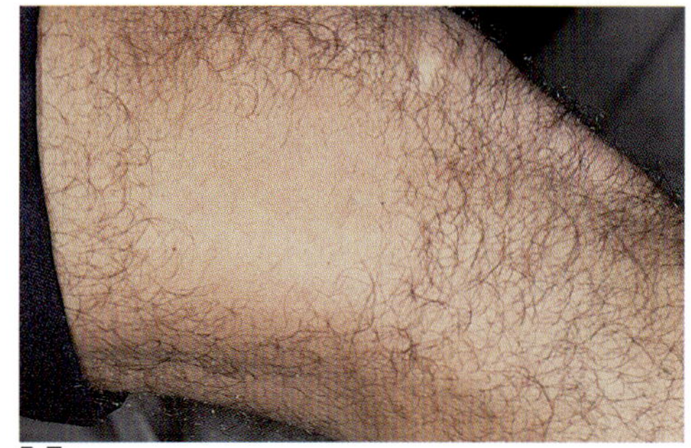
5.7c ■

Specific forms of alopecia areata are recognized: 1) Ophiasis (derived from Greek for snake) is the band-like loss along the periphery of the temporal-occipital scalp (Figures 5.6a,b), 2) diffuse alopecia areata, perhaps the most difficult to diagnose clinically, represents areas where hair remains thin and short probably due to recurrent episodes of loss and regrowth, 3) reticular alopecia areata represents persistent multiple patches of loss.

Lesions of alopecia areata may occur on other sites as isolated phenomena or in association with scalp lesions. Such sites include eyebrows, upper and lower eyelashes (Figure 5.7a), the beard area (Figure 5.7b) and trunk or limbs (Figure 5.7c). Nail involvement (Figures 5.8a,b) is usually associated with widespread alopecia areata. The initial hair regrowth after an episode of alopecia areata is often white (Figure 5.9) due to a delay in the remelanization of affected hairs. Interestingly, the last hairs to be affected in an attack of alopecia areata are white hairs, explaining how scalps can appear to become white overnight (Figure 5.10). The association between Down's syndrome and alopecia areata is shown in Figures 5.11a,b.

The prevalence of alopecia areata is approximately one per 1,000 of the general population. However,

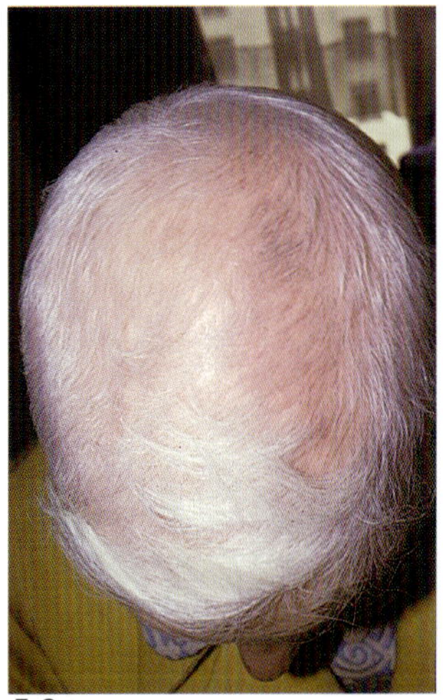
5.9

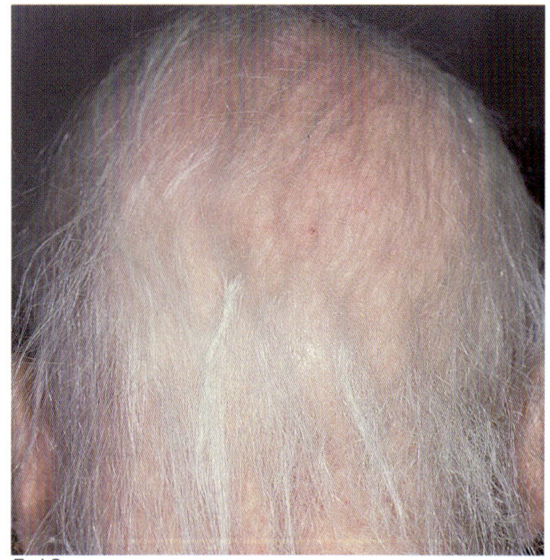
5.10

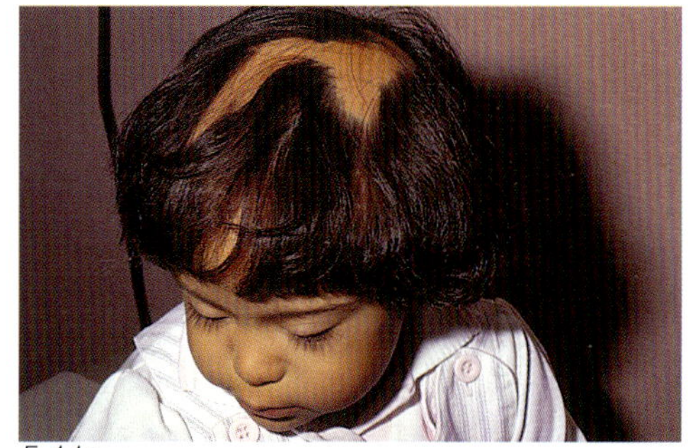
5.11a →

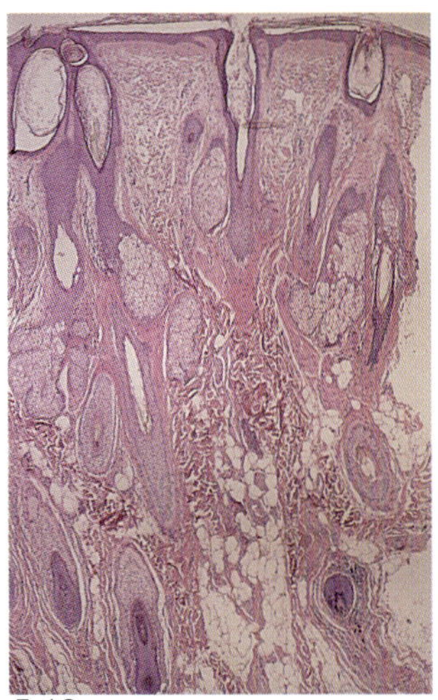
5.12a →

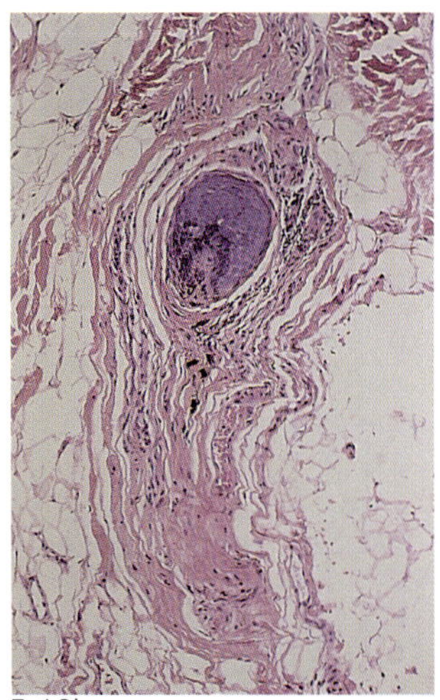
5.12b ■

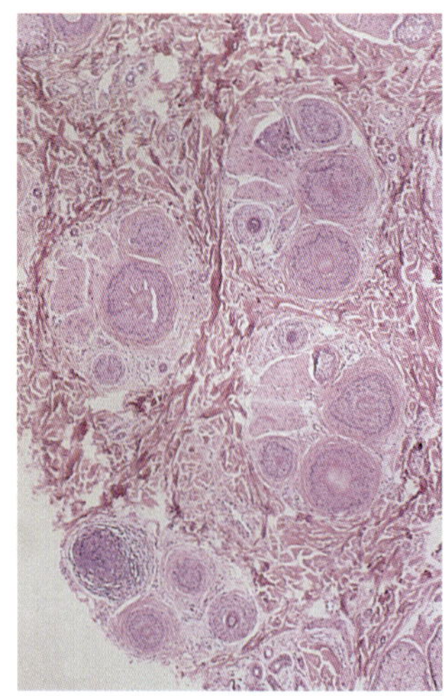
5.13a →

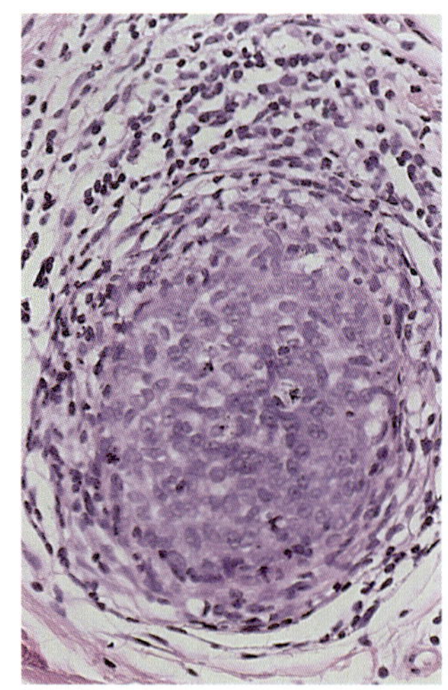
5.13b →

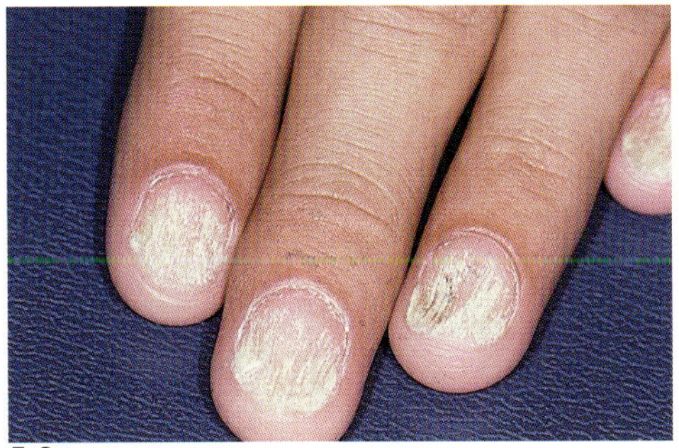
5.8a →

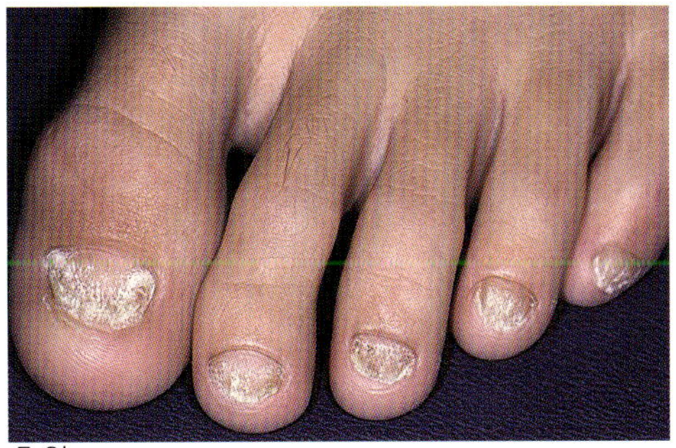
5.8b ■

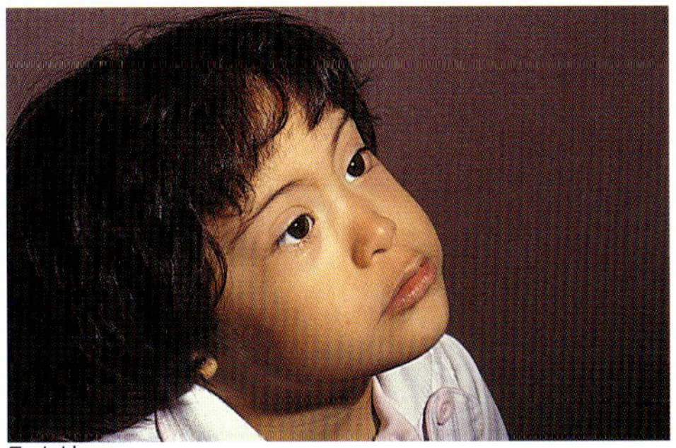
5.11b ■

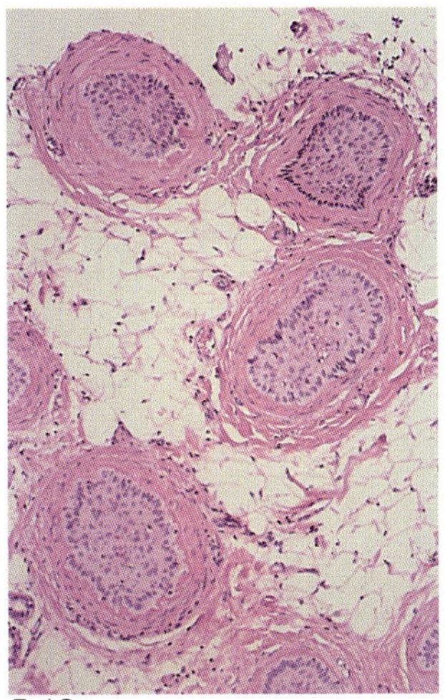
5.13c →

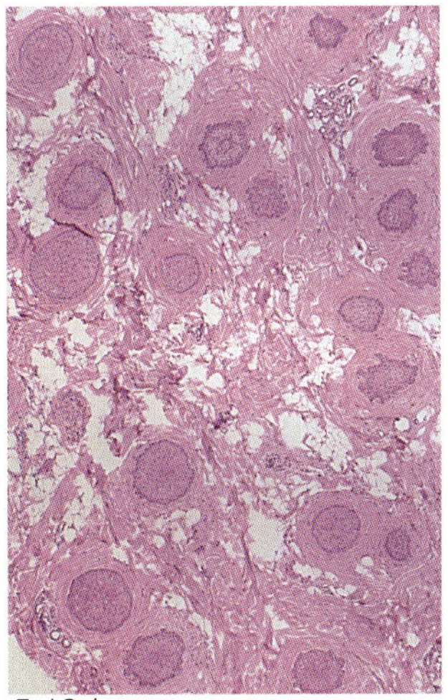
5.13d ■

5.7
Alopecia areata:

a. Patchy alopecia affects both eyelids here.

b. Alopecia areata: Several patches of alopecia in the beard area.

c. Alopecia areata: Circular patch of alopecia on right thigh.

5.8
Alopecia areata: Nail dystrophy:

a. Severe fingernail dystrophy with pitting and vertical ridging.

b. Severe toenail dystrophy with pitting and vertical ridging.

5.9
Alopecia areata: Initial hair regrowth following alopecia totalis is white in color.

5.10
Alopecia areata: Sudden onset of diffuse alopecia has affected the black hairs only, and has left the grey hairs intact, explaining how in rare instances the scalp hair can appear to become white overnight.

5.11
Alopecia areata: Down's syndrome:

a. Large area of alopecia areata on scalp.

b. Characteristic facial appearance.

5.12
Scalp biopsy: Histopathology of alopecia areata: Vertical section:

a. Lymphocytic infiltration around one hair bulb. LM x 40.

b. Lymphocytes are clustered around hair bulb and extend into follicular stela. LM x 100.

5.13
Scalp biopsy: Histopathology of alopecia areata: Horizontal section:

a. Lower dermis: Decreased numbers of terminal hairs, with increased follicular stelae, and increased catagen hairs. LM x 40.

b. Lower dermis: Lymphocytes are swarming around the hair bulb and also penetrating the bulb. LM x 300.

c. Lower dermis: Increased catagen hairs are present. LM x 100.

d. Upper dermis: Increased telogen hairs and increased vellus hairs are present. LM x 40.

it has been stated that one out of every 100 Americans will develop a patch of alopecia areata by age 50 years. The long-term prognosis in patients with alopecia areata is impossible to predict in any given case. It is discouraging to note that in one study in which 230 patients were followed for up to 20 years, 100% were found to have relapses. Poor prognosis has been assigned to patients who develop disease before puberty, who have multiple episodes of loss, who have the ophiasis type distribution of loss and who have an associated atopic diathesis. The greater the extent of hair loss and the longer the duration of activity the poorer the prognosis as well. In the USA, following Ikeda's classification, roughly 75% of cases have uncomplicated alopecia areata, with onset peaking in the third and fourth decades of life, 20% have associated atopic diseases with an earlier onset, often in childhood, and 5% have associated autoimmune or endocrine diseases, with onset peaking in middle age. Alopecia totalis may occur in some 6% of the uncomplicated cases, 10% of the autoimmune cases, and 40% or more of the atopic cases.

Histopathology

Scalp biopsies taken in the acute stage of alopecia areata show a characteristic cluster of lymphocytes around follicular bulbs, the so-called "swarm of bees" (Figures 5.12a,b). Some histiocytes may be present. The infiltrate can involve the bulb, the adjacent suprabulbar portion of the hair shaft, or the follicular streamer (stelae). The process usually involves terminal hairs but can affect "vellus" hairs as well. Some of the affected hairs remain in the anagen stage, but many cycle through catagen into a premature telogen phase. Miniaturization of affected follicles can occur. These changes can be enumerated on horizontal sections of scalp biopsies (Figures 5.13a,b,c,d) which show a decreased anagen to telogen ratio, resulting from a marked increase in telogen hairs, and often in catagen hairs also. The terminal to "vellus" hair ratio is decreased and even reversed by the increased numbers of miniaturized hairs. Inflammatory changes in the mid and upper dermis are generally not prominent unless many "vellus" hairs are affected by the disease. Dense scarring is not seen.

Investigation and Diagnosis

The history of an abrupt onset of patchy hair loss, the lack of infection, scaling, black dots and irregular stubble, the presence of exclamation point hairs of uniform length, and a slick, depressed feel to the affected area of scalp, are all suggestive of the diagnosis of alopecia areata. The absence of scarring excludes cicatricial alopecia, and traction alopecia can usually be excluded if there is no evidence of stressed hair styling; however, traction alopecia involving scalp hair margins and ophiasis sometimes have overlapping features, and trichotillomania or tinea capitis have been known to co–exist with alopecia areata. Potassium hydroxide preparations of broken off hairs, and fungal cultures, are often useful. However, in some cases scalp biopsies are necessary for definitive diagnosis.

Differential Diagnosis

Causes of patchy alopecia which may cause diagnostic confusion here include tinea capitis, traction alopecia, trichotillomania, aplasia cutis, congenital triangular alopecia, loose anagen syndrome, familial focal alopecia, pressure alopecia, secondary syphilis, tick bite alopecia, and pseudopelade.

Treatment

Patch type alopecia areata can be treated with a wait-and-see approach and many lesions will regrow spontaneously. Mosaic forms or steadily enlarging patches may respond to topical corticosteroid applications or intralesional steroids. Topical short-contact anthralin therapy may be useful in children who cannot tolerate injections. Topical minoxidil solution is sometimes helpful. Immunosuppressive therapy with systemic corticosteroids can be combined with minoxidil for short periods in treating widespread alopecia. Other systemic agents such as cyclosporin may have a dramatic effect, but the effects are usually temporary and side effects can be dangerous. Immunotherapy with a topical sensitizer such as diphencyprone is sometimes successful, but again the effects are often transient and the therapy should still be considered experimental; its side effects may be poorly tolerated. ■

Suggested Reading

Beard, H.O.: "Social and psychological implications of alopecia areata." *J Am Acad Dermatol* 1986;14:697–700.

Bystryn, J.C., Orentreich, N., Stengel, F.: "Direct immunofluorescence studies in alopecia areata and male pattern alopecia." *J Invest Dermatol* 1979;73:317–320.

Caserio, R.J.: "Treatment of alopecia areata with squaric acid dibutylester." *Arch Dermatol* 1987;123:1036–1041.

Claudy, A.L., Gagnaire,D.: "PUVA treatment of alopecia areata." *Arch Dermatol* 1983;119:975–978.

Cole, G.W., Herzlinger, D.: "Alopecia universalis in identical twins." *Int J Dermatol* 1984;23:283.

Crosby, D.L., Gammon, W.R.: "Seasonal alopecia areata with atopy." *J Am Acad Dermatol* 1989;21:806–807

Daman, L.A., Rosenburg, W., Drake, L.: "Treatment of alopecia areata with dinitrochlorobenzene." *Arch Dermatol* 1978;114:1036–1038.

Duvic, M., Hordinsky, M.K., Fiedler, V.C., et al.: "HLA–D locus associations in alopecia areata: DRW52A may confer disease resistance." *Arch Dermatol* 1991;127:64–68

Elieff, D., Sundby, S., Kennedy, W., et al.: "Decreased sweat–gland number and function in patients with alopecia areata." *Br J Dermatol* 1991;125:130–135.

Fiedler, V.C., Wendrow, A., Szpunar, G.J., et al.: "Treatment–resistant alopecia areata. Response to combination therapy with minoxidil plus anthralin." *Arch Dermatol* 1990;126:756–759.

Fiedler, V.C.: "Alopecia areata. A review of therapy, efficacy, safety, and mechanism." *Arch Dermatol* 1992;128:1519–1529.

Fiedler–Weiss, V.C.: "Topical minoxidil solution (1% and 5%) in the treatment of alopecia areata." *J Am Acad Dermatol* 1987;16:745–748.

Fiedler–Weiss, V.C., Buys, C.M.: "Evaluation of anthralin in the treatment of alopecia areata." *Arch Dermatol* 1987;123:1491–1493.

Frentz, G., Thomsen, K., Jakobsen, B.K., et al.: "HLA–DR4 in alopecia areata (letter)." *J Am Acad Dermatol* 1986;14:129–130.

Friedmann, P.S.: "Alopecia areata and auto–immunity." *Br J Dermatol* 1981;105:153–157.

Galbraith, G.M.P., Theirs, B.H., Vasily, D.B., et al.: "Immunological profiles in alopecia areata." *Br J Dermatol* 1984;110:163–170.

Gilhar, A., Krueger, G.G.: "Hair growth in scalp grafts from patients with alopecia areata and alopecia universalis grafted onto nude mice." *Arch Dermatol* 1987;123:44–50.

Gupta, A.K., et al.: "Oral cyclosporine for the treatment of alopecia areata." *J Am Acad Dermatol* 1990;22:242–250.

Happle, R., Klein, M., Macher, E.: "Topical immunotherapy changes the composition of peribulbar infiltrate in alopecia areata." *Arch Dermatol Res* 1986;278:214–218.

Healy, E., Rogers, S.: "PUVA treatment for alopecia areata—does it work? A retrospective review of 102 cases." *Br J Dermatol* 1993;129:42–44.

Hordinsky, M.K., Hallgren, H., Nelson, O., et al.: "Suppressor cell number and function in alopecia areata." *Arch Dermatol* 1984;120:188–194.

Hordinsky, M.K., Hollgren, H., Nelson, D., et al.: "Familial alopecia areata. HLA antigens and autoantibody formation." *Arch Dermatol* 1984;120:464–468.

Hordinsky, M.K.: "Alopecia areata." In: *Disorders of Hair Growth. Diagnosis and Treatment,* Olsen, E.A. (Ed.). New York: McGraw–Hill 1994, 195–222.

Ikeda, T.: "A new classification of alopecia areata." *Dermatologica* 1965;131:421– 445.

Jillson, O.F.: "Alopecia. I. Alopecia areata." *Cutis* 1983;31:262,266,269–273.

Kern, F., Hoffmann, W.H., Hambrick, G.W., et al.: "Alopecia areata. Immunologic studies and treatment with prednisone." *Arch Dermatol* 1973;107:407–412.

Khoury, E.L., Price, V.H., Abdel-Salam, M.M., et al.: "Topical minoxidil in alopecia areata: No effect on the perifollicular lymphoid infiltration." *J Invest Dermatol* 1992;99:40–47.

Klaber, M.R., Munro, D.D.: "Alopecia areata: immunofluorescence and other studies." *Br J Dermatol* 1978;99:383–386.

Lowry, M., Ledoux-Carbusier, M., Achten, G., et al.: "Clinical and immunologic response to isoprinosine in alopecia areata." *J Am Acad Dermatol* 1985;12:78–84.

MacDonald-Hull, S., Nutbrown, M., Pepall L., et al.: "Immunohistologic and ultrastructural comparison of the dermal papilla and hair follicle bulb from "active" and "normal" areas of alopecia areata." *J Invest Dermatol* 1991;96:673–681.

Majewski, B.B.J., Koht, M.S., Taylor, D.R., et al.: "Increased ratio of helper to suppressor T cells in alopecia areata." *Br J Dermatol* 1984;110:171–175.

Messenger, A.G., Bleehen, S.S.: "Alopecia areata: Light and electron microscope pathology of the regrowing white hair." *Br J Dermatol* 1984;110:155–162

Messenger, A.G., Slater, D.N., Bleehen, S.S.: "Alopecia areata alterations in the hair growth cycle and correlation with follicular pathology." *Br J Dermatol* 1986;114:337–347.

Michie, H.J., Jahoda, C.A.B., Oliver, R.F., et al.: "The DEBR rat: an animal model of human alopecia areata." *Br J Dermatol* 1991;125:94–100.

Mitchell, A.J., Douglass, M.C.: "Topical photochemotherapy for alopecia areata." *J Am Acad Dermatol* 1985;12:644–649.

Mitchell, A.J., Krull, E.A.: "Alopecia areata: pathogenesis and treatment." *J Am Acad Dermatol* 1984;11:763–775.

Muller, S.A., Winkelmann, R.K.: "Alopecia areata: An evaluation of 736 patients." *Arch Dermatol* 1963;88:290–297.

Nelson, D.A., Spielvogel, R.L.: "Alopecia areata." *Int J Dermatol* 1985;24:26–34.

Olsen, E.A.: "Systemic steroids with or without 2% topical minoxidil in the treatment of alopecia areata." *Arch Dermatol* 1992;128:1467–1473.

Price, V.H.: "Topical minoxidil (3%) in extensive alopecia areata including long–term efficacy." *J Am Acad Dermatol* 1987;16:737–744.

Shapiro, J.: "Alopecia areata. Update on therapy." *Dermatologic Clinics* 1993;11:35– 46.

Swanson, N.A., Mitchell, A.J., Leahy, M.S., et al.: "Topical treatment of alopecia areata: contact allergies vs primary irritant therapy." *Arch Dermatol* 1981;117:384–387.

Todes-Taylor, N., Tumer, R., Wood, G.S., et al.: "T cell subpopulations in alopecia areata." *J Am Acad Dermatol* 1984;11:216–223.

Tosti, A., Baradazzi, F., Guerra, L.: "Alopecia totalis: Is treating nonresponder patients useful?" *J Am Acad Dermatol* 1991;24:455–456.

Tosti, A., Colombate, S., Caponeri, G.M., et al.: "Ocular abnormalities occurring with alopecia areata." *Dermatologica* 1985;170:69–73.

Tosti, A., DePadova, M.P., Minghetti, G., et al.: "Therapies versus placebo in the treatment of patchy alopecia areata." *J Am Acad Dermatol* 1986;15:209–210.

Unger, W.P., Schemmer, R.J.: "Corticosteroids in the treatment of alopecia areata." *Arch Dermatol* 1978;114:1486–1490.

Valsecchi, R., Bontempelli, M., Vicari, O.: "Peripheral T cell subsets in patients with alopecia areata in different clinical phases." *Dermatologica* 1985;171:170–174.

Valsecchi, R., Vicari, O., Frigent, A., et al.: "Familial alopecia areata – genetic susceptibility or coincidence?" *Acta Derm Venereol* (Stockh) 1985;2:65,175–177.

Walker, S.A., Rothman, S.: "Alopecia areata. A statistical study and consideration of endocrine influences." *J Invest Dermatol* 1950;14:403–413.

Whiting, D.A.: "Treatment of alopecia areata." *Cutis* 1987;40:247–250.

Cicatricial Alopecia

Definition

Cicatricial alopecia results from permanent destruction and fibrosis of hair follicles. It is usually circumscribed but may be widespread.

Etiology

Many congenital and acquired causes of cicatricial alopecia are listed in Table 6.1. Those illustrated here include aplasia cutis (Figure 6.1), nevus sebaceous (Figures 6.2a,b), verrucous epidermal nevus (Figure 6.3), epidermolysis bullosa dystrophica (Figure 6.4), facial hemiatrophy (Figure 6.5), acne keloidalis (Figure 6.6), dissecting folliculitis (Figure 6.7), tinea capitis (Figures 6.8a,b), angiosarcoma (Figures 6.9a,b), neoplastic infiltration (Figures 6.10a,b), folliculitis decalvans (Figures 6.11a,b), pseudopelade (Figures 6.12a,b, 6.13a,b), erosive pustular dermatosis (Figure 6.14), follicular mucinosis (Figures 6.15a,b), Graham-Little syndrome (Figure 6.16), lichen planus (Figures 6.17a,b), lichen planopilaris (Figures 6.18a,b), discoid lupus erythematosus (Figures 6.19a,b,c), necrobiosis lipoidica (Figures 6.20a,b), and scleroderma en coup de sabre (Figure 6.21).

Clinical Description

In many cases the scarring may be circumscribed and obvious. In others scarring may be more subtle and diffuse, as in marginal alopecia caused by continuous traction from stressed hair styles. Changes on the scalp may include folliculitis, follicular plugging, absent follicular orifices, scaling, telangiectasia and broken hairs. Associated lesions may be present elsewhere on the skin and mucous membranes, including ears, nails and mouth. Easily extractable anagen hairs with an intact external root sheath may be found on the scalp in active areas of lichen planopilaris, discoid lupus erythematosus, and pseudopelade, and in some cases twisted hairs are found. A specific diagnosis may be possible in active disease, but in burnt out cases the permanent destruction of follicles and associated scarring can look the same regardless of the cause, and a definite diagnosis is difficult or impossible.

Folliculitis Decalvans:
Crops of follicular pustules surround multiple, slowly-expanding, round or oval areas of alopecia in the scalp (Figures 6.11a,b) and sometimes in the pubic and axillary areas.

Discoid Lupus Erythematosus:
Erythema, atrophy and telangiectasia occur in discoid lupus erythematosus. Scaly crusts with follicular spines like carpet tacks attached to the under surface are more likely to occur well inside the affected bare patches rather than at their margins (Figures 6.19a,b,c). The active lesions may be sensitive and pruritic.

Lichen Planopilaris:
Bare, white patches may be seen in the early stages of lichen planopilaris

(continued)

Table 6.1 Causes of cicatricial alopecia*

Developmental and inherited defects		Aplasia cutis Chondrodysplasia punctata Cutis verticis gyrata Darier's disease Eccrine hamartoma Epidermal nevi	Epidermolysis bullosa Facial hemiatrophy Hair–follicle hamartoma Hypotrichosis congenita Ichthyosis – sex–linked recessive	Incontinentia pigmenti Keratosis pilaris atrophicans Neurofibromatosis Polyostotic fibrous dysplasia Porokeratosis of Mibelli Scarring follicular keratosis
Infections	**Bacterial**	Acne keloidalis Acne necrotica Carbuncle Furuncle	Dissecting cellulitis of scalp (perifolliculitis) Folliculitis Tuberculosis	Leprosy Lupoid sycosis Syphilis
	Fungal	Favus Kerion Mycetoma	Tinea capitis – other inflammatory forms	
	Protozoal	Leishmaniasis	Onchocerciasis	
	Viral	Herpes zoster	Varicella	
Exogenous traumatic damage		Burns Chemical burns	Insect bites Mechanical trauma	Radiodermatitis
Neoplasms		Angiosarcoma Basal–cell epithelioma Benign lymphoplasias Cylindroma	Dermatofibrosarcoma protruberans Malignant lymphomas Malignant melanoma Metastatic tumors	Nerve–sheath myxoma Reticulosis Squamous–cell carcinoma Syringoma
Dermatoses	**Syndromes:**	Alopecia parvimacularis	Graham-Little syndrome	Lipedematous alopecia
	Diseases:	Amyloidosis Cicatricial pemphigoid Eosinophilic cellulitis Erosive pustular dermatosis Follicular mucinosis Giant cell arteritis Folliculitis decalvans	Granuloma annulare Lichen sclerosus et atrophicus Lichen simplex with scarring from excoriations, dermatitis artifacta, prurigo, etc. Pseudopelade	Lupus erythematosus Scleroderma Sjogren's syndrome

*After Rook, A., Dawber, R.: Diseases of the Hair and Scalp (2nd Ed). Oxford: Blackwell Scientific Publications, 1991:334–369.

but prominent follicular hyperkeratosis is usually present around residual terminal hairs, with varying degrees of erythema, scaling, and telangiectasia (Figures 6.18a,b). Itching may be present. Follicular hyperkeratosis may also be present on chest, back and limbs.

Pseudopelade of Brocq:
Classic pseudopelade affects whites and orientals. It presents with patchy areas of alopecia, with irregular extensions into the surrounding scalp hair, which contain smooth, white areas of skin devoid of erythema, scaling or pores, the so-called "footprints in the snow" (Figures 6.12a,b). A second form of pseudopelade involves the central scalp of black females of 20 to 40 years of age. A large patch of alopecia with smooth skin, a few pores and hairs, and indistinct margins occurs with asymmetrical pseudopod-like extensions (Figure 6.13a). The belief that this type of change was entirely due to hotcombing has not been substantiated, and some regard it as a form of follicular degeneration. A third form of pseudopelade affecting whites and orientals has been described. It produces an elliptical area of hair loss over the central scalp, with mild perifollicular inflammation (Figure 6.13b). The end stages of folliculitis decalvans, discoid lupus erythematosus, lichen planopilaris, and
(continued on page 46)

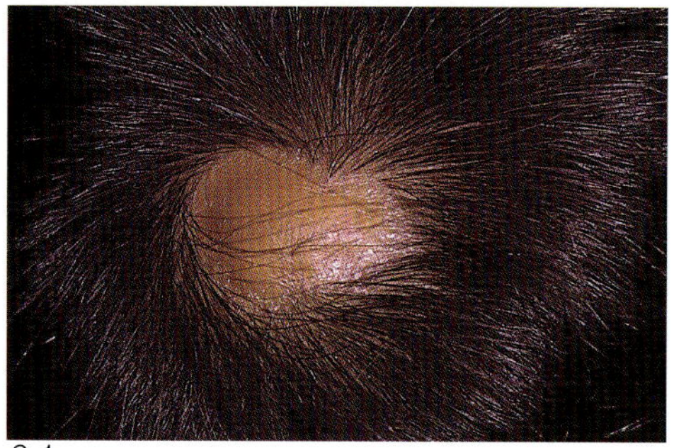
6.1

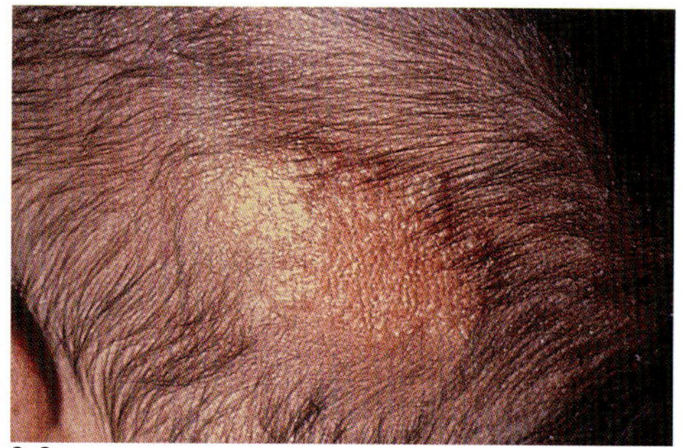
6.2a ➔

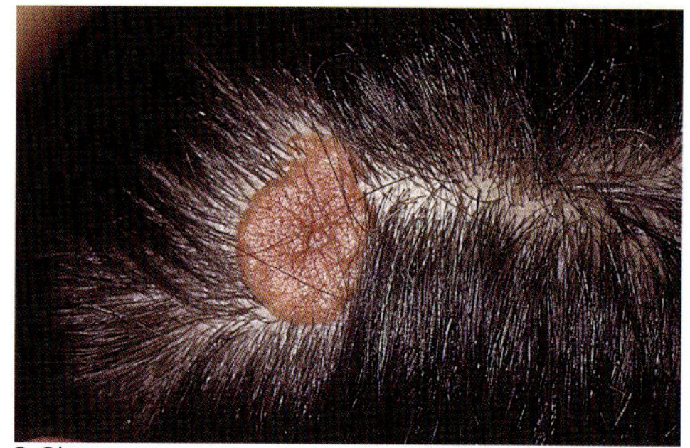
6.2b ■

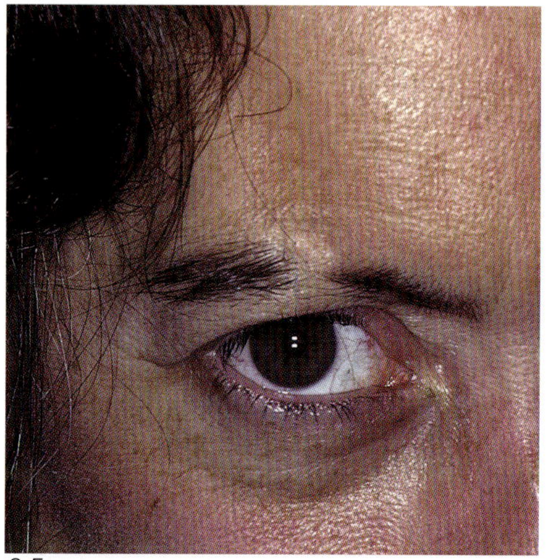
6.5

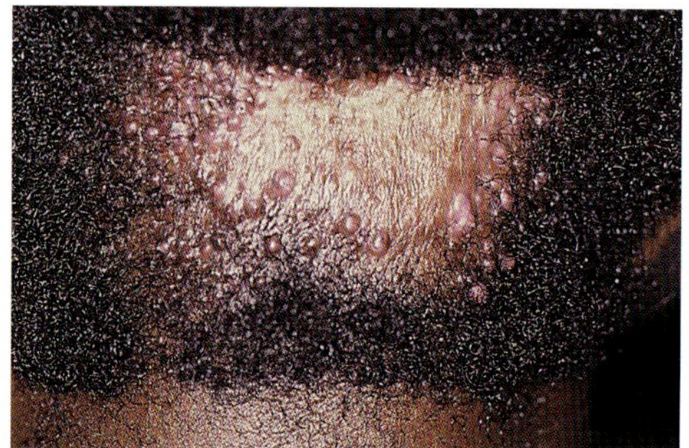
6.6

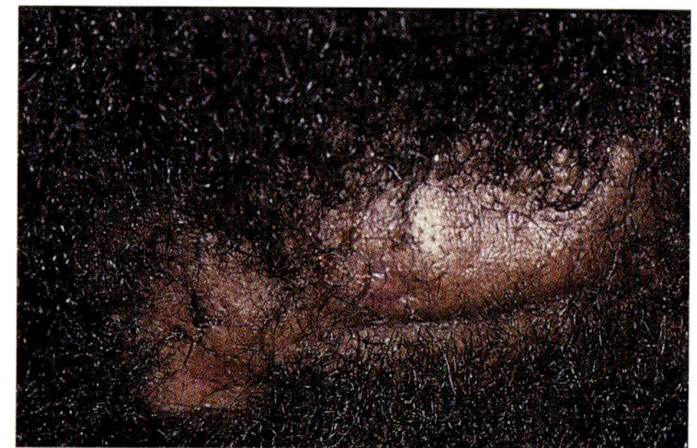
6.7

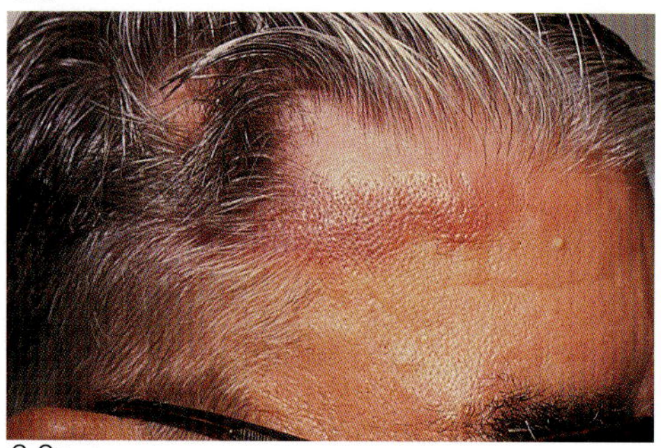
6.9a ➔

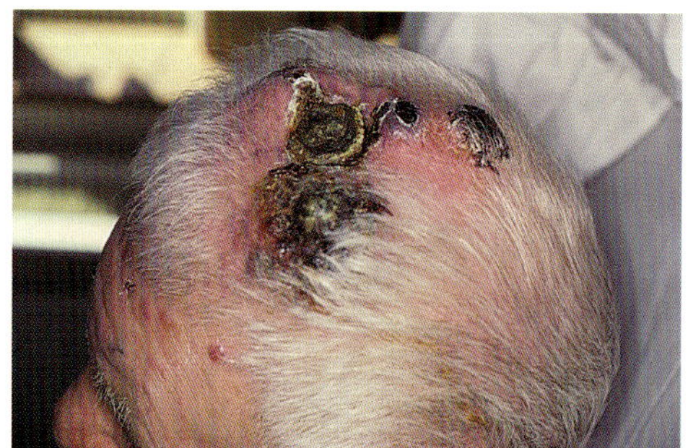
6.9b ■

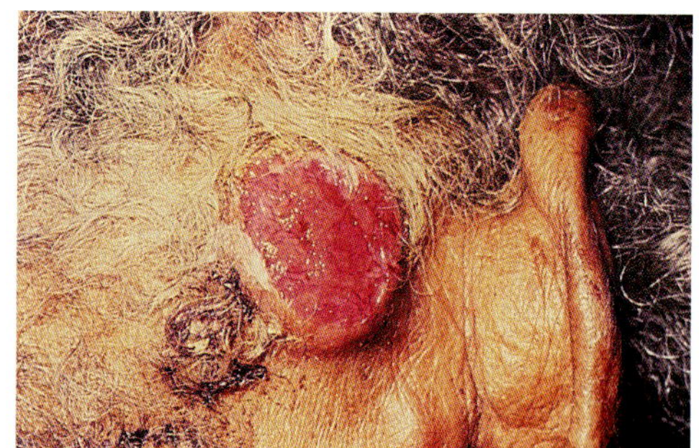
6.10a ➔

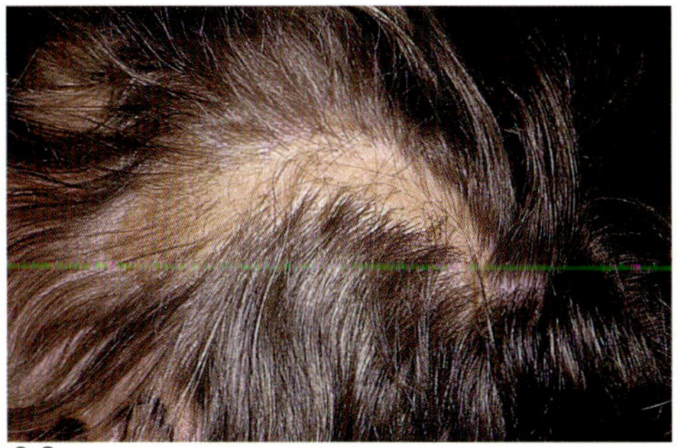
6.3

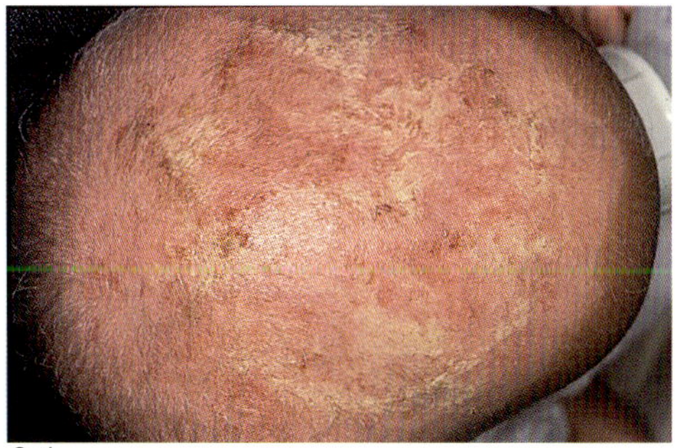
6.4

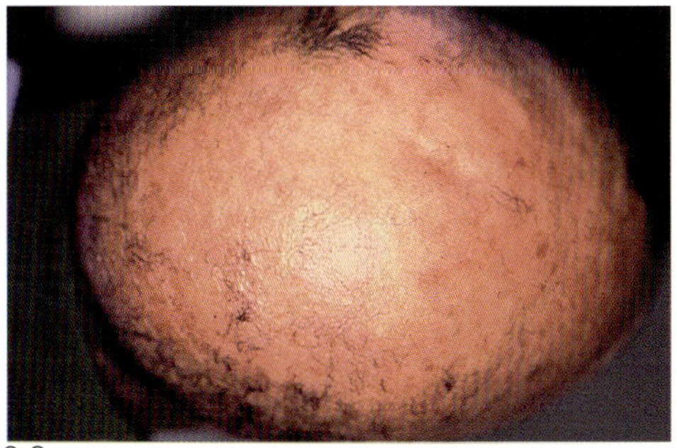
6.8a →

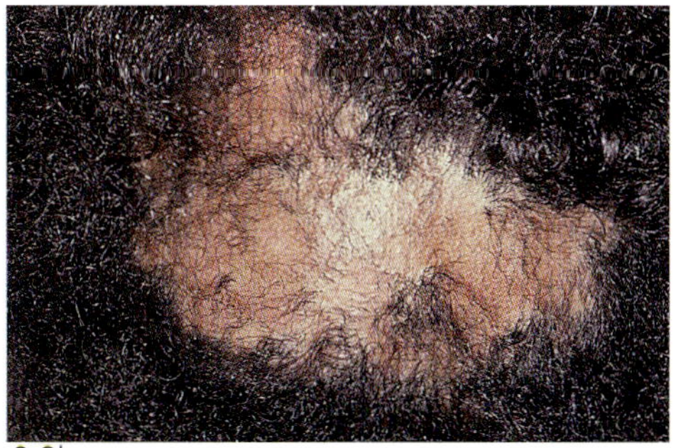
6.8b ■

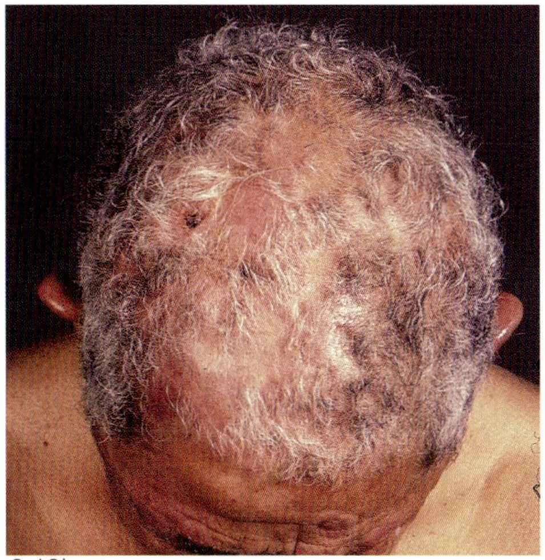
6.10b ■

6.1
Aplasia cutis with hairless area of scarring.

6.2
Nevus sebaceus:

a. In infancy, due to maternal androgens, the lesion is temporarily prominent as a salmon colored, hairless patch.

b. In adults the lesion has become permanently prominent due to androgen production with puberty. Lesion is raised and hairless.

6.3
Verrucous epidermal nevus: A hairless, linear area of verrucous skin is present.

6.4
Epidermolysis bullosa dystrophica: Recurrent blistering has led to cicatricial alopecia.

6.5
Facial hemiatrophy: Atrophic scarring extends from hairline across eyebrow onto cheek.

6.6
Acne keloidalis: Severe, scarring alopecia with keloidal papules.

6.7
Perifolliculitis capitis abscessens et suffodiens: Dissecting folliculitis has caused scarring, alopecia, and discharging sinuses.

6.8
Scarring caused by tinea capitis:

a. Favus: Cicatricial alopecia following favus is generalized and severe. *(Courtesy of H. Francois Jordaan, M.Med.)*

b. Kerion: Patchy cicatricial alopecia is common after a severe kerion.

6.9
Angiosarcoma:

a. Early lesion.

b. Late lesion. (Courtesy of *H. Francois Jordaan, M. Med.*)

6.10.
Neoplastic cicatricial alopecia:

a. Metastatic neoplasm: Cicatricial alopecia is associated with a large metastatis from carcinoma of the breast. *(Courtesy of H. Francois Jordaan, M. Med.)*

b. Cutaneous T–cell lymphoma: Multiple, destructive lesions of mycosis fungoides have caused a severe cicatricial alopecia. *(Courtesy of H. Francois Jordaan, M. Med.)*

6.11
Folliculitis decalvans:

a. Cicatricial alopecia is seen with sparse hairs, some of which show folliculitis.

b. Extensive infection from folliculitis decalvans has led to severe scarring. Some active folliculitis is visible.

6.12
Pseudopelade:

a. Classical pseudopelade in Caucasians shows an irregular scarring with pod-like extensions.

b. The pale areas here are called "foot-prints in the snow" and are typical of pseudopelade.

6.13
Pseudopelade:

a. Centrally located pseudopelade is relatively common in middle-aged black females and can cause extensive symmetrical alopecia of the vertex.

b. Central pseudopelade can also occur in Caucasians.

6.14
Erosive pustular dermatosis of the scalp: This rare condition is chronic and resistant to antibiotics and may show extensive confluent pustules or more scattered folliculitis and pustulation as seen here. An underlying tinea capitis was eventually demonstrated in this case.

6.15
Follicular mucinosis:

a. A patch of alopecia is present in center of moustache area.

b. Skin biopsy: Histopathology: Horizontal section: Mucinous changes are present in external root sheath of hair follicle. LM x 400.

6.16
Graham-Little syndrome: Severe scarring alopecia on scalp in child, with loss of eyebrows associated with follicular plugging.

6.17
Lichen planus:

a. Lichenoid papules on the scalp.

b. Classical reddish-brown lesions on the shin.

6.18
Lichen planopilaris:

a. Central, cicatricial alopecia is surrounded by hairs with prominent follicular scales, and erythema.

b. Old lesions show severe scarring with prominent hairs around the margins of the scar.

6.19
Discoid lupus erythematosus:

a. Active disease has caused a large area of cicatricial alopecia with telangiectasia, atrophy and follicular plugging. *(Reprinted with permission, Whiting, D.A., The Diagnosis of Alopecia, Current Concepts, Upjohn, 1990.)*

b. An older lesion shows central activity with uninvolved area of old scarring around the periphery. *(Reprinted with permission, Whiting, D.A., The Diagnosis of Alopecia, Current Concepts, Upjohn, 1990.)*

c. An old, scarred lesion with dilated pores and follicular plugging.

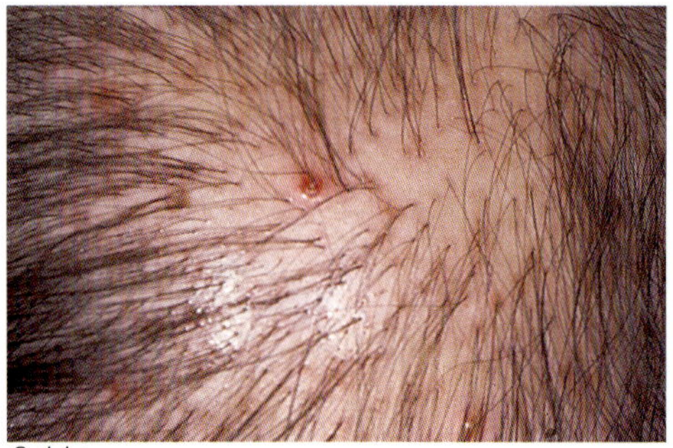
6.11a →

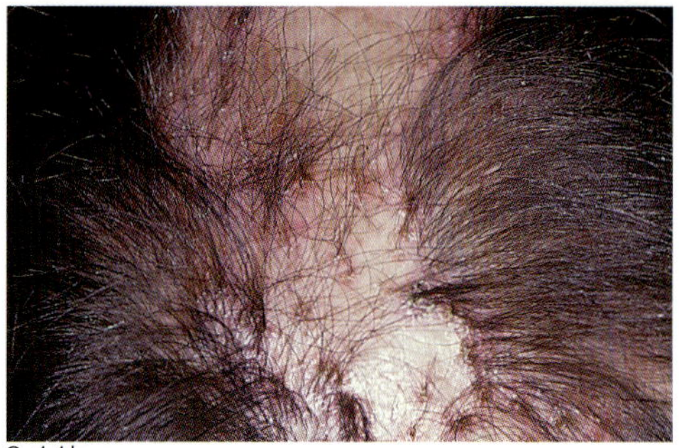
6.11b ■

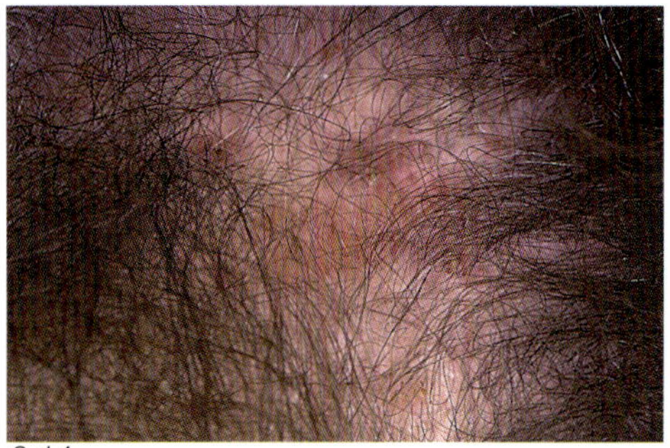
6.14

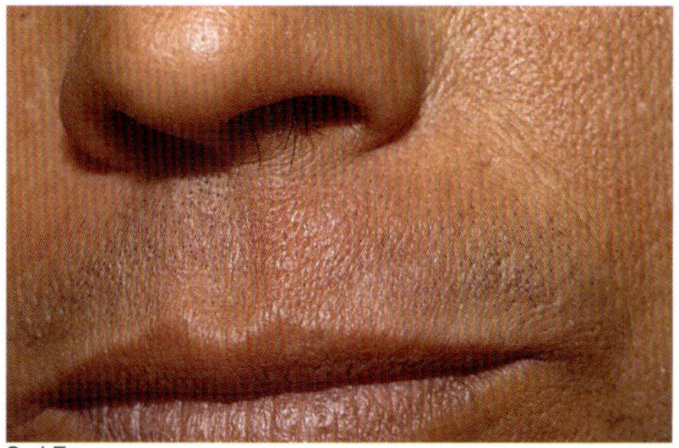
6.15a →

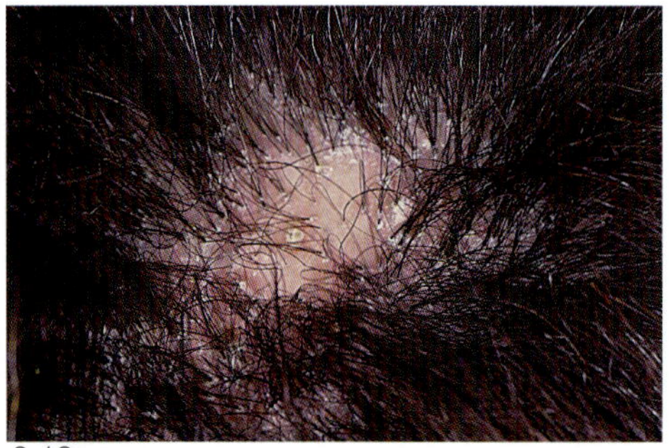
6.18a →

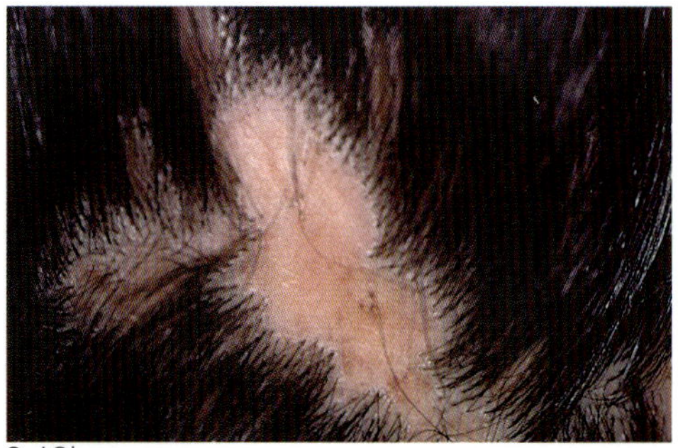
6.18b ■

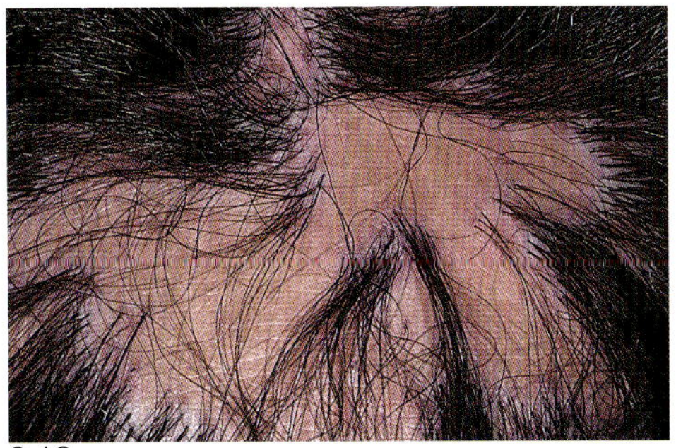

6.12a →

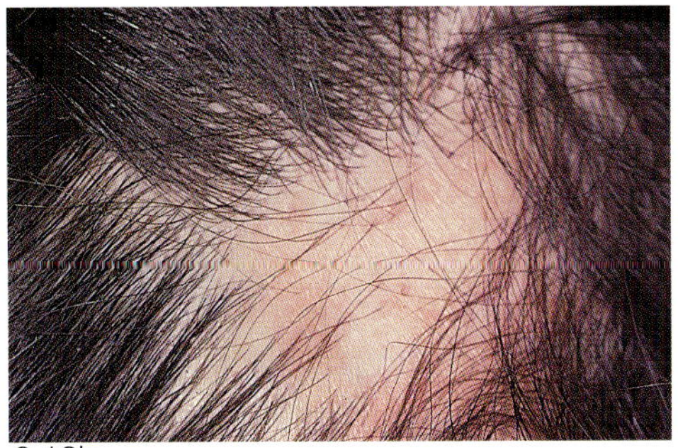

6.12b ■

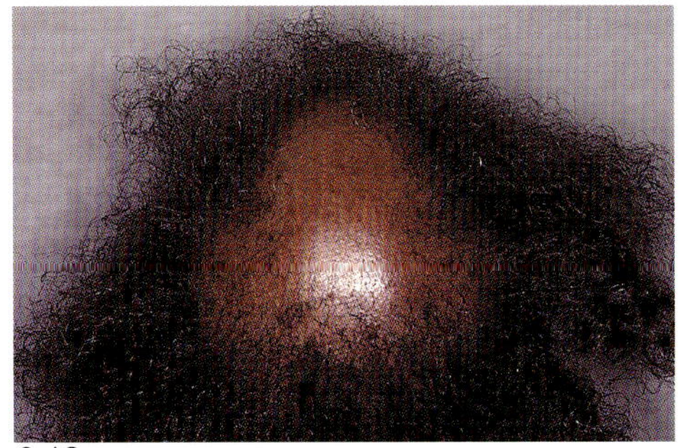

6.13a →

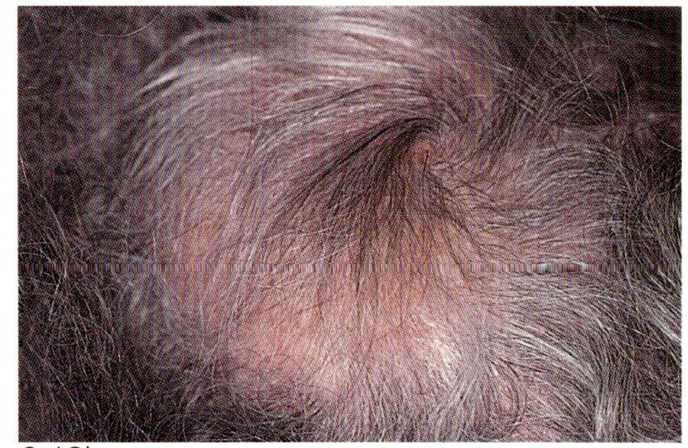

6.13b ■

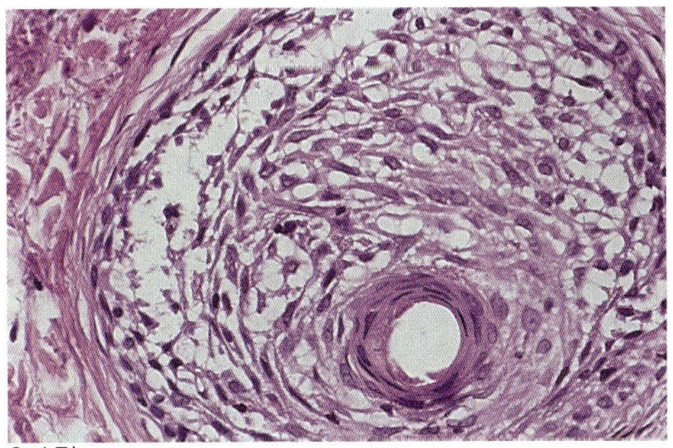

6.15b ■

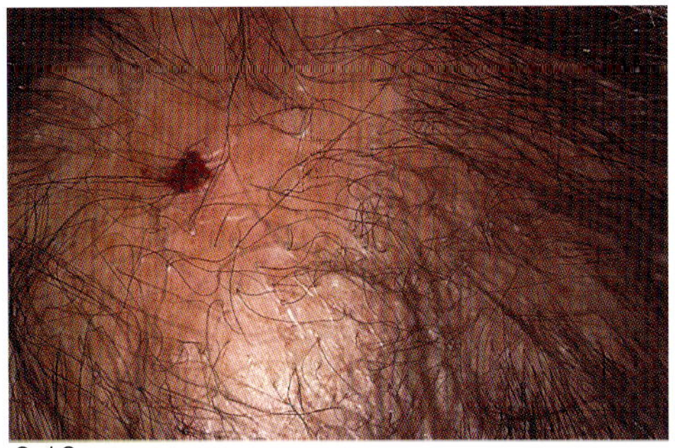

6.16

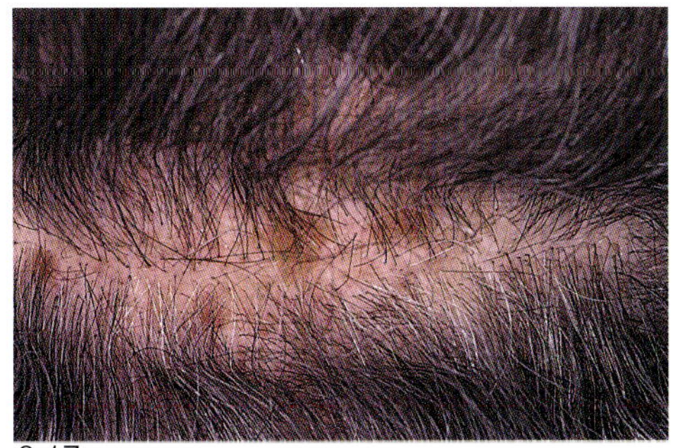

6.17a →

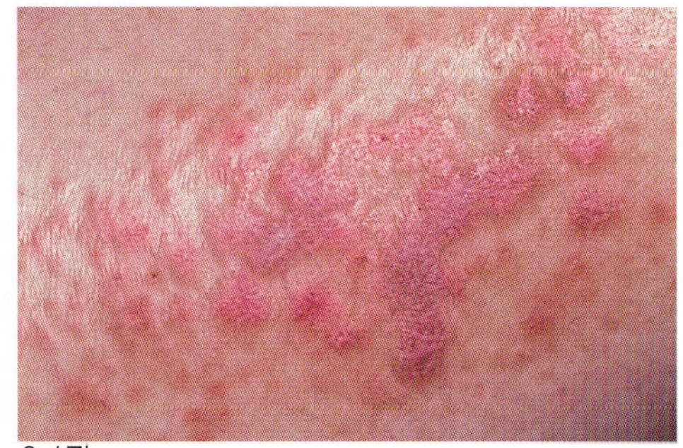

6.17b ■

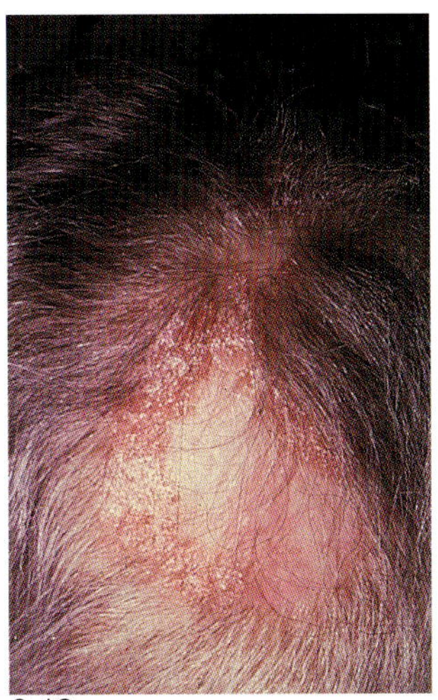

6.19a →

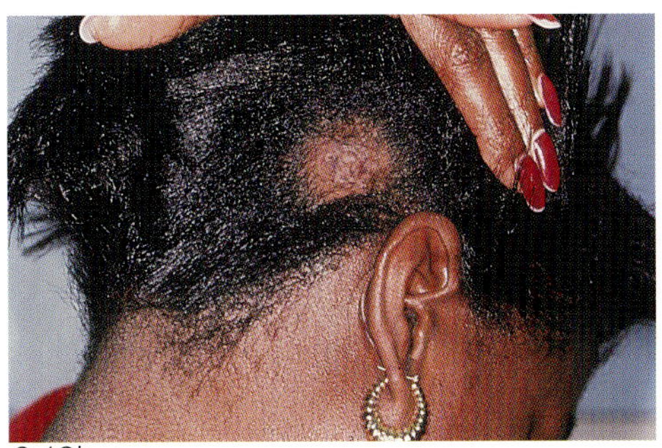

6.19b →

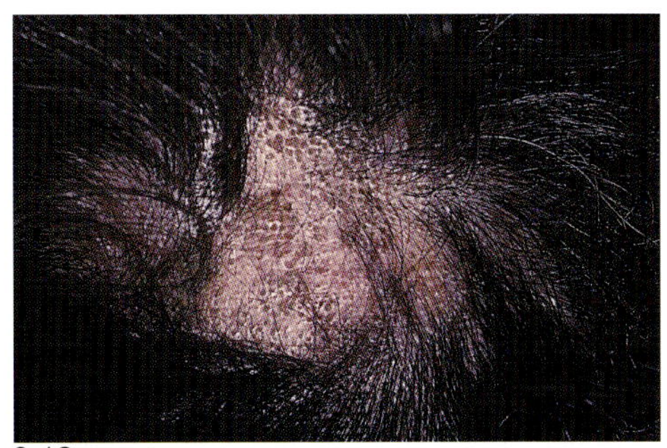

6.19c ■

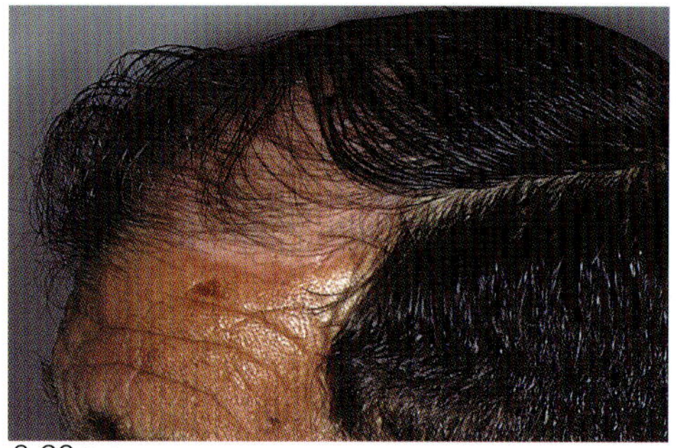
6.20a ➔

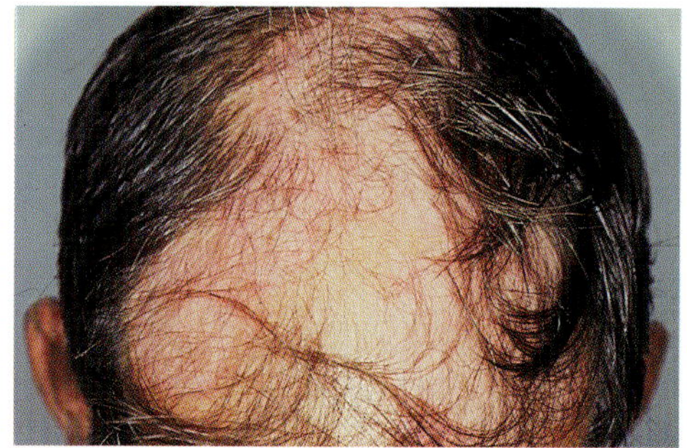
6.20b ■

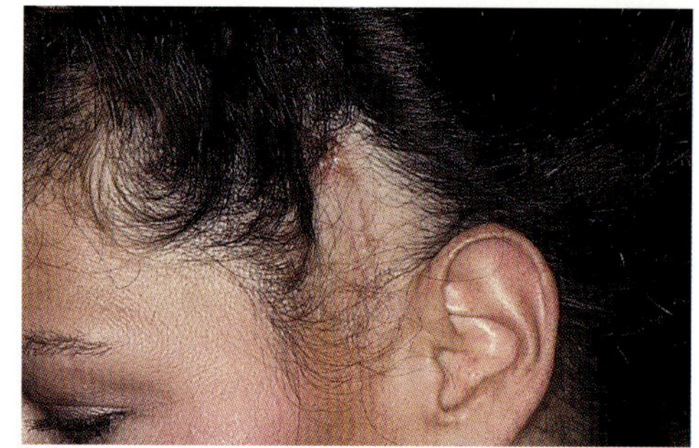
6.21

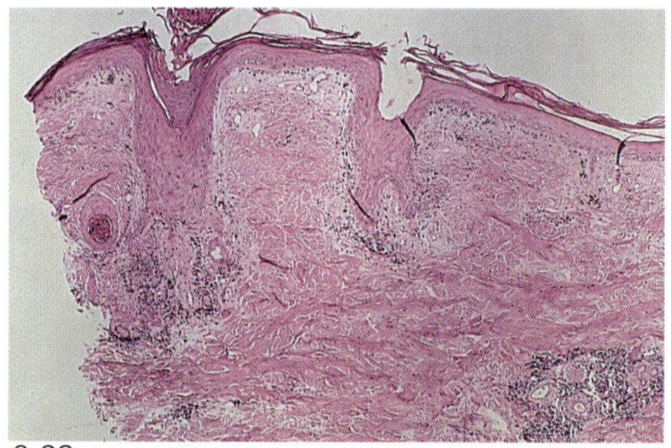
6.23a ➔

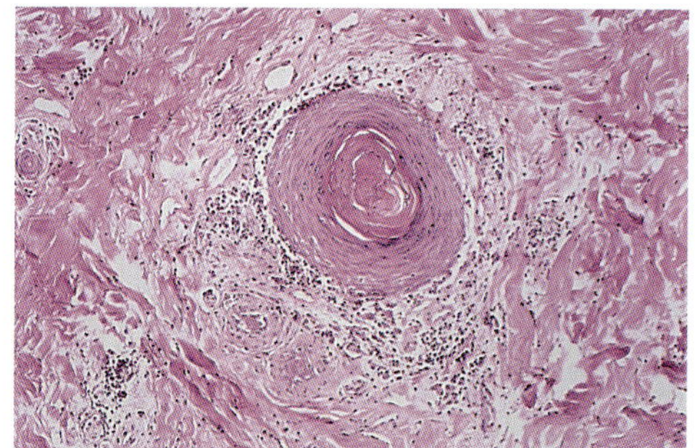
6.23b ➔

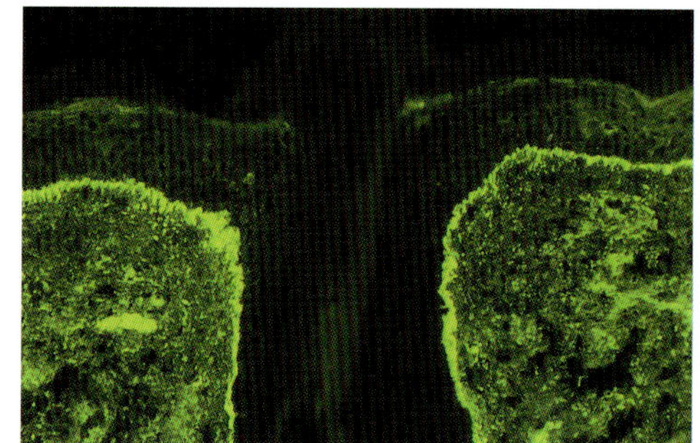
6.23c ■

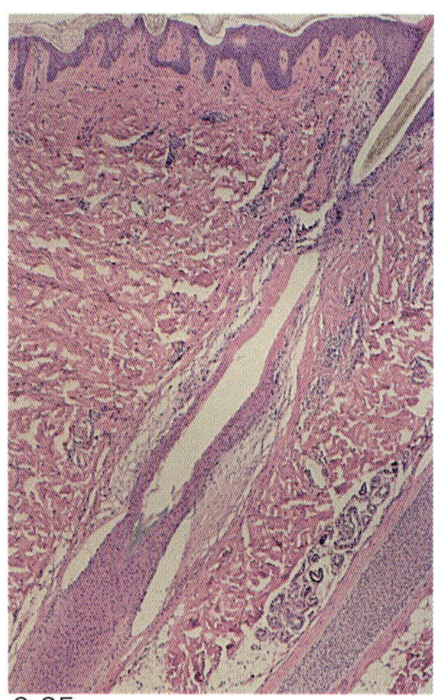
6.25a ➔

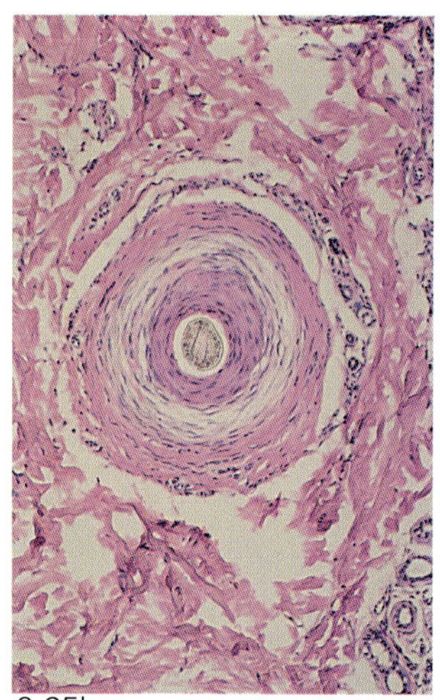
6.25b ■

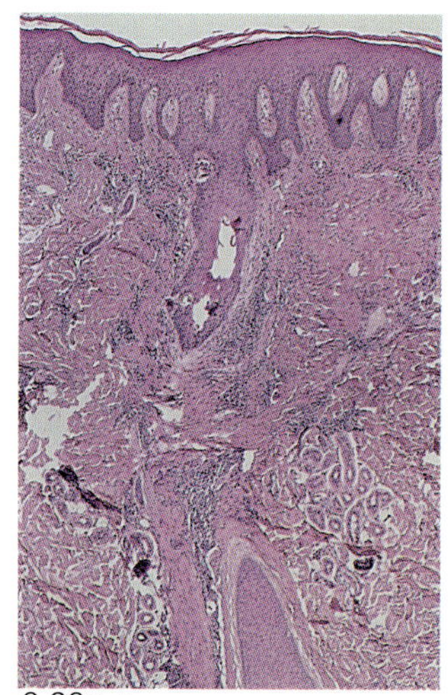
6.26a ➔

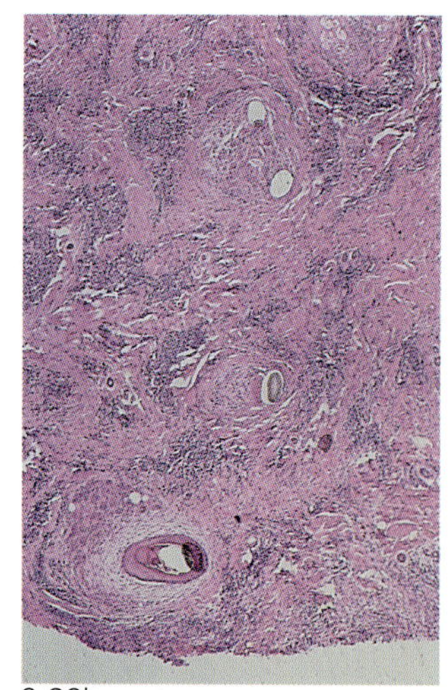
6.26b ■

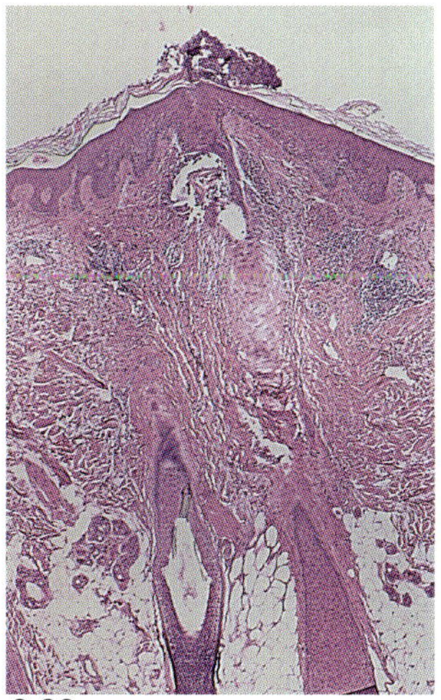

6.22a →

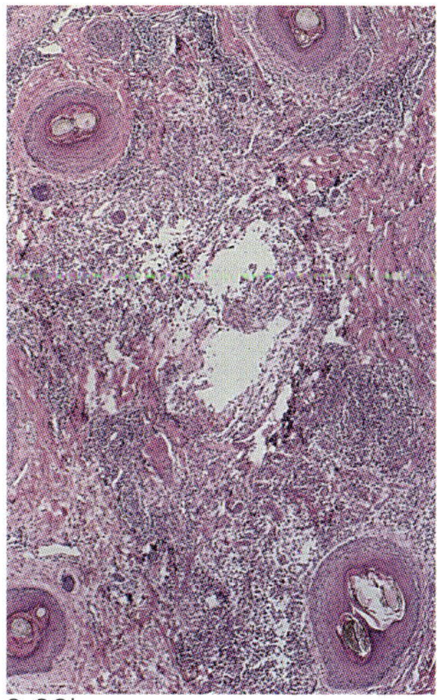

6.22b ■

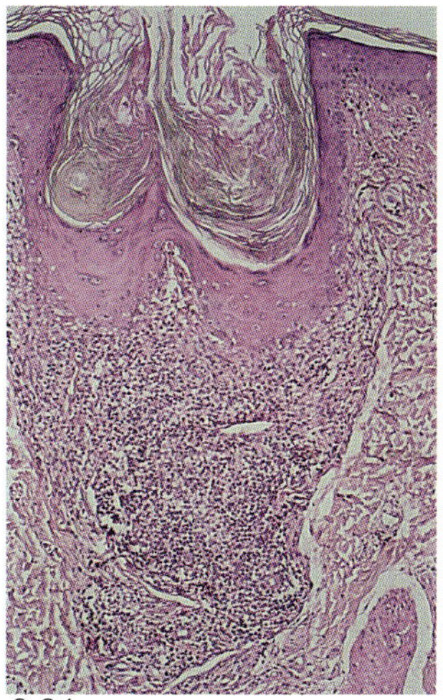

6.24a →

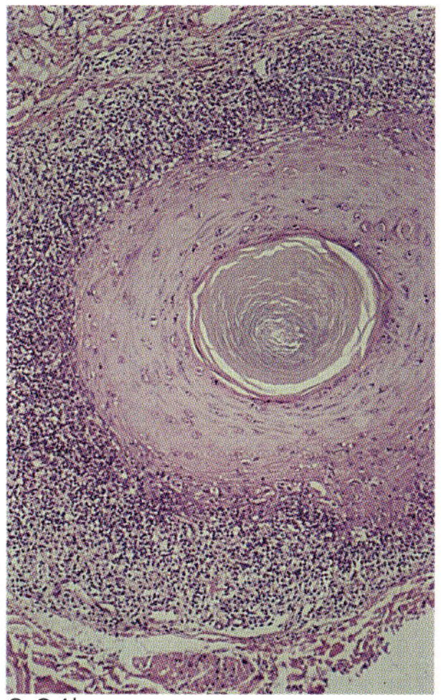

6.24b →

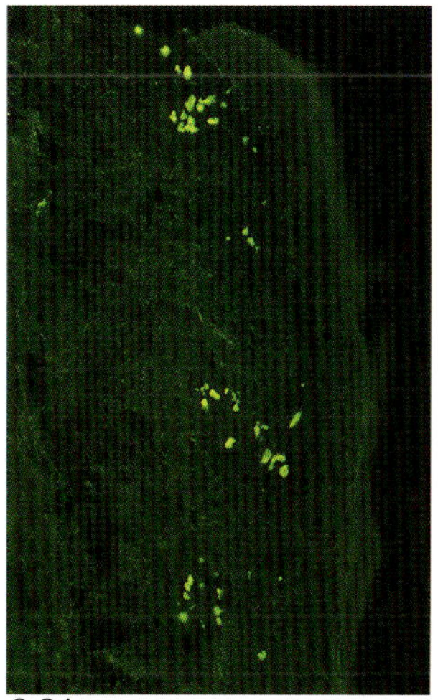

6.24c ■

6.20
a,b. Necrobiosis lipoidica (discoid granulomatosis of Miescher): An old name for this was annular sarcoid, and annular erythema and scarring are visible here.

6.21
Scleroderma en coup de sabre: Involves left temple and cheek.

6.22
Scalp biopsy: Histopathology of folliculitis decalvans:

a. Vertical section: Upper dermis: Severe folliculitis with pustulation in the upper follicle is surrounded by acute and chronic inflammatory changes and scarring. LM x 40.

b. Horizontal section: Upper dermis: A severe pustular folliculitis involves upper follicles with acute and chronic inflammatory changes and scarring. LM x 40.

6.23
Scalp biopsy: Histopathology of lupus erythematosus:

a. Vertical section: A lymphoid infiltration around follicles and sweat glands is associated with a thin epidermis. LM x 40.

b. Horizontal section: Upper dermis: An affected hair follicle is surrounded by a lichenoid infiltration of lymphocytes, which is invading the basal layer of the epithelium. LM x 100.

c. Immunofluorescence: A solid, bright layer at the dermo-epidermal junction is stained by immunoglobulin G, the so–called lupus band.

6.24
Scalp biopsy: Histopathology of lichen planopilaris:

a. Vertical section: Lower dermis: A typical, lichenoid infiltrate of lymphocytes and histocytes surrounds the base of a hair follicle. LM x 100.

b. Horizontal section: Upper dermis: A dense lichenoid infiltrate of lymphocytes and histocytes surrounds the external root sheath of the follicle and invades the basal layer. LM x 100.

c. Immunofluorescence: Many cytoid bodies line the affected hair follicle.

6.25
Scalp biopsy: Histopathology of pseudopelade:

a. Vertical section: Perifollicular fibrosis is present around mid follicle with minimal inflammatory infiltrate. LM x 40.

b. Horizontal section: Perifollicular fibrosis with minimal inflammatory change. LM x 100.

6.26
Scalp biopsy: Histopathology of acne keloid:

a. Vertical section: Marked, perifollicular fibrosis and chronic, inflammatory changes are present around both upper and lower follicles. LM x 40.

b. Horizontal section: Marked perifollicular fibrosis is seen around extruded hair fragments and hair follicles. A high density of lymphocytes, histocytes, and plasma cells with foreign body giant cells is present in the areas of inflammation. LM x 40.

pseudopelade are similar, with scarring alopecia and loss of pore markings. Some feel that pseudopelade represents a late stage of lichen planopilaris, but others regard its early stages as distinctive.

Histopathology

A scalp biopsy should be done in all cases of cicatricial alopecia, and in general a definitive diagnosis is possible if the lesion is active.
Active folliculitis decalvans shows upper and mid follicular inflammation with acute and chronic inflammatory cells, and follicular rupture and destruction (Figures 6.22a,b).
Active discoid lupus erythematosus shows follicular plugging, epidermal atrophy, hydropic degeneration of the basal layer, and a deeply extending lymphocytic infiltrate which is often periadnexal (Figures 6.23a,b,c).
Early lichen planopilaris shows follicular plugging, perifollicular hypergranulosis, a perifollicular lichenoid infiltrate, basal layer destruction and cytoid bodies (Figures 6.24a,b,c).
End stage lesions of all three show the same extensive scarring and follicular loss seen in pseudopelade (Figures 6.25a,b).
Immunofluorescence is useful for diagnosing discoid lupus under these circumstances (Figure 6.23c), but the findings in lichen planopilaris are inconsistent (Figure 6.24c). The histology of acne keloidalis shows folliculitis, follicular rupture, foreign body reaction and fibrosis around both upper and lower follicles (Figures 6.26a,b).

Investigation and Diagnosis

Scalp biopsies are mandatory in cicatricial alopecia. Bacterial, fungal, or viral cultures may be indicated. Appropriate laboratory and radiological investigations may be required.

Differential Diagnosis

Old lesions of alopecia areata and focal familial alopecia may be confused with pseudopelade.
Histological examination is necessary although this may be inconclusive in regressing alopecia areata. Familial focal alopecia shows telogen arrest with no inflammation or scarring.

Treatment

The treatment of cicatricial alopecia depends on the cause and whether active disease is present. Tumors can be excised, preferably by simple ellipse and suture. Infections are treated appropriately. Discoid lupus erythematosus and lichen planopilaris may be amenable to treatment with topical, intralesional or systemic corticosteroids and/or antimalarials. End stage scarring can be excised by ellipse or scalp reduction, or hair transplants may be inserted. ■

Suggested Reading

Altman, J., Perry, H.O.: "The variations and course of lichen planus." *Arch Dermatol* 1961;84:179–191.

Braun-Falco, O., Bergner, T., Heilgemier, G.P.: "Pseudopelade alopecia." *Hautarzt* 1989;40:77–83.

Braun-Falco, O., Imai, S., Schmoeckel, C., et al.: "Pseudopelade of Brocq." *Dermatologica* 1986;172:18–23.

Brozena, S.J., Cohen, L.E., Fenske, N.A.: "Folliculitis decalvans – response to rifampin." *Cutis* 1988;42:512–515.

Bulengo-Ransby, S.M., Headington, J.T.: "Pseudopelade of Brocq in a child." *J Am Acad Dermatol* 1990;23:944–945.

Elston, D.M., Bergfeld, W.F.: "Cicatricial alopecia (and other causes of permanent alopecia)." In: *Disorders of Hair Growth. Diagnosis and Treatment,* Olsen, E.A. (Ed.). New York: McGraw–Hill 1994, 285–313.

Feldman, S.: "Lichen planus et acuminatus atrophicans: folliculitis decalvans et lichen spinulosis of Little." *Arch Dermatol Syphilol* 1936;34:378–397.

Ioannides, D., Bystryn, J.C.: "Immunofluorescence abnormalities in lichen planopilaris." *Arch Dermatol* 1992;128:214–216.

Little, E.G.: "Lichen spinulosis et folliculitis decalvans: report of a case." *Proc R Soc Med* 1921;14:67–68.

Lo Presti, P., Papa, C.M., Kligman, A.M.: "Hot comb alopecia." *Arch Dermatol* 1968;98:234–238.

Matla, M., Kibbi, A-G., Khattar, J., et al.: "Lichen planopilaris: A clinicopathologic study." *J Am Acad Dermatol* 1990;22:594–598.

Mehregan, A.H.: "Histopathology of alopecia." *Cutis* 1978;21:249–253.

Mehregan, D.A., Van Hale, H.M., Muller, S.A.: "Lichen planopilaris: Clinical and pathological study of forty-five patients." *J Am Acad Dermatol* 1992;27:935–942.

Nayar, M., Schomberg, K., Dawber, R.P.R., et al.: "A clinicopathological study of scarring alopecia." *Br J Dermatol* 1993;128:533–536.

Nicholson, A.G., Hewland, C.C., Bull, R.H., et al.: "Chemically induced cosmetic alopecia." *Br J Dermatol* 1993;128:537–541.

Pinkus, H.: "Alopecia." *Int J Dermatol* 1980;19:245–253.

Pinkus, H.: "Alopecia mucinosa. Additional data in 1983." *Arch Dermatol* 1983;119:698–699.

Price, V.H.: "Management of hair problems." *Int J Dermatol* 1979;18:95–103.

Prieto, J.G.: "Pseudopelade of Brocq: its relationship to some forms of cicatricial alopecia and to lichen planus." *J Invest Dermatol* 1955;24:223–335.

Rook, A., Dawber, R.: *Diseases of the Hair and Scalp* (2nd ed.). Oxford: Blackwell Scientific Publications, 1991:334–369.

Sachs, W., DeOreo, G.: "Lichen planopilaris." *Arch Dermatol Syphilol* 1942;45:1081– 1093.

Silvers, D.N., Katz, B.E., Young, A.W.: "Pseudopelade of Brocq is lichen planopilaris: Report of four cases that support this nosology." *Cutis* 1993;51:99–105.

Singh, O.P., Konwar, A.J.: "Lichen planus in India: an appraisal of 441 cases." *Int J Dermatol* 1976;15:752–756.

Snyder, R.A., Crain, W.R., McNutt, N.S.: "Alopecia mucinosa. Report of a case with diffuse alopecia and normal-appearing scalp skin." *Arch Dermatol* 1984;120:496- 498.

Sperling, L.C., Sau, P.: "The follicular degeneration syndrome in black patients." *Arch Dermatol* 1992;128:68–74.

Traupe, H., Happle, R.: "Alopecia ichthyotica. A characteristic feature of congenital ichthyosis." *Dermatologica* 1983;167:280–282.

Trozak, D.J., Wood, C.: "Occult eccrine sweat duct hamartoma and cicatricial scalp alopecia." *Cutis* 1984;34:475–477.

Vakilzadeh, F., Brocker, E.B.: "Syringolymphoid hyperplasia with alopecia." *Br J Dermatol* 1984;110:95–101.

Van Scott, E.J., Reinertson, R.P.: "Detection of radiation effects on hair roots of the human scalp." *J Invest Dermatol* 1957;29:205–212.

Wilson, C.L., Burge, S.M., Dean, D., et al.: "Scarring alopecia in discoid lupus erythematosus." *Br J Dermatol* 1992;126:307–314.

Trichotillomania

Definition

Trichotillomania is an abnormal compulsion to pull out hair.

Etiology

Trichotillomania is caused by an underlying emotional problem or by definite mental disorder. In children, the underlying problem is often easy to discern; causes include lack of attention, sibling rivalry, divorced parents, unhappiness at school, and learning disabilities; in some children, mental retardation may be a factor. In adults, the disease is far more intractable and is usually due to a severe psychological disorder, often a monosymptomatic hypochondriacal psychosis, or to definite mental deficiency.

Clinical Description

Trichotillomania affects twice as many females as males, except under the ages of six where the sex ratio is three males to one female. The peak incidence is in the 2-6 year age group, and the child may develop the habit subconsciously; it may replace thumb sucking. The more severe form affects mainly females from adolescence onwards, with the peak age of 11-17 years. It usually affects the scalp hair (Figures 7.1a,b, 7.2a,b) but is sometimes seen in the eyebrows and upper eyelashes (Figures 7.3a,b). The eyelashes on the lower lids are not affected since they are difficult to grasp with the fingers. In the great majority of cases the patient's own hair is pulled out, but in some cases hair is extracted from other people. The affected patches may be small or large, and are often asymmetrical. Severe cases of so-called tonsure alopecia affect both sides of the scalp in a symmetrical pattern (Figure 7.2a). An irregular stubble is felt in the affected areas. The hairs are seen to be broken off at different lengths (Figure 7.2b), unlike the more uniform exclamation mark hairs of alopecia areata or the black dots of endothrix tinea capitis. Pale, tapered, newly growing anagen hairs may be present in relatively large numbers. The underlying scalp is normal, and is not smooth and atrophic as in alopecia areata or inflamed and scaly as in tinea capitis. Hair pull tests may be positive or negative but as a rule do not hurt the patient.

(continued)

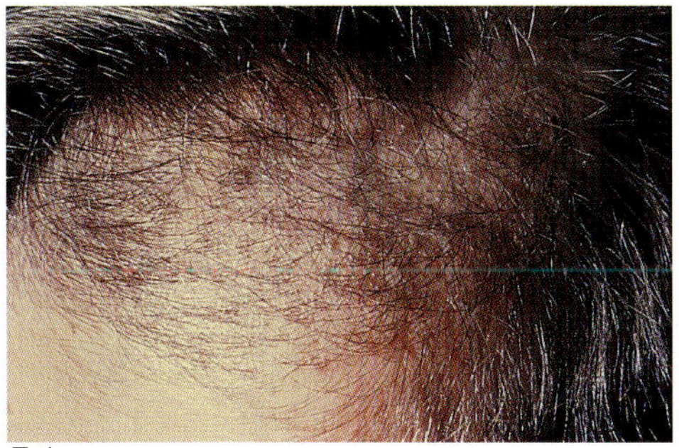

7.1a ➔

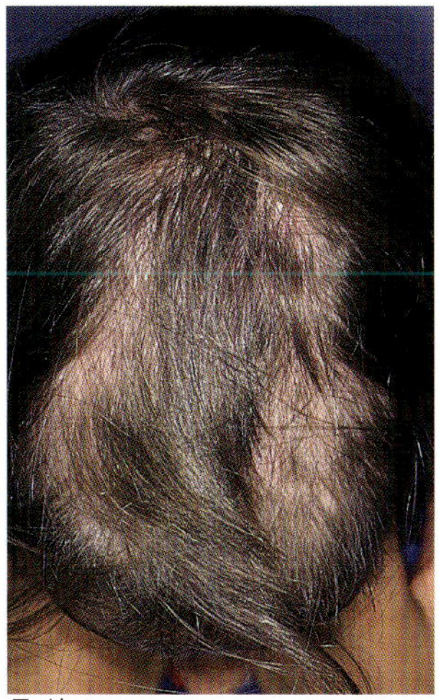

7.1b ■

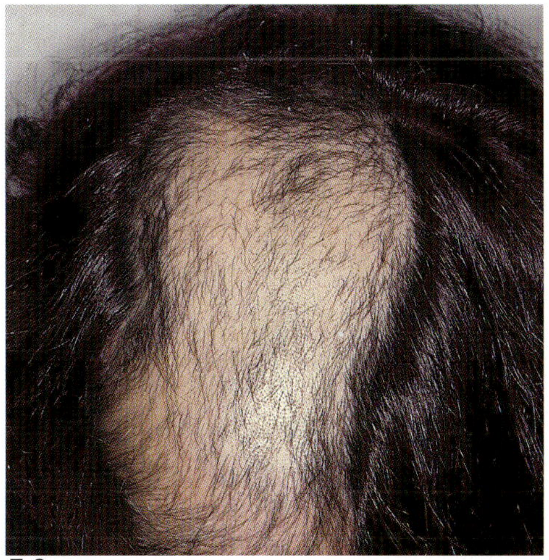

7.2a ➔

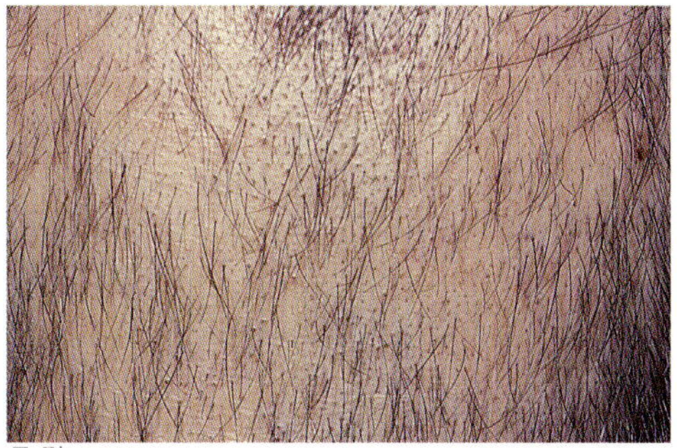

7.2b ■

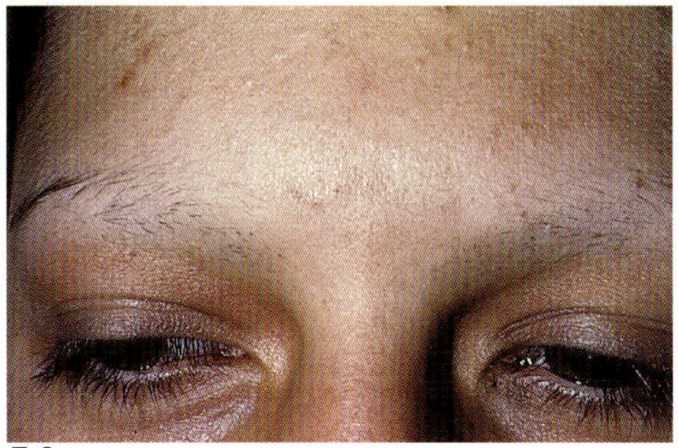

7.3a ➔

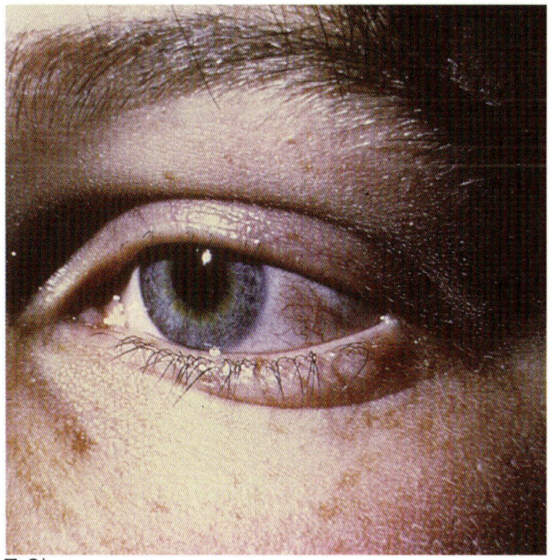

7.3b ■

7.1
Trichotillomania:

a. A single patch of trichotillomania is shown here. The hair is broken off at irregular lengths. The scalp shows no inflammatory change, scaling or atrophy.

b. Several patches of trichotillomania are present here.

7.2
Tonsure trichotillomania:

a. A large bare patch at center of head.

b. A closer inspection shows hairs broken off at different lengths with a normal underlying scalp.

7.3
Trichotillomania:

a. Trichotillomania of eyebrows.

b. Trichotillomania of eyelashes characteristically involving only the upper eyelashes because the lower eyelashes are difficult to grasp. *(Reprinted with permission, Whiting, D.A., The Diagnosis of Alopecia, Current Concepts, Upjohn, 1990.)*

Histopathology

Scalp biopsies usually show a lack of inflammatory change. Follicular plugging and pigment casts are often present, and sometimes perifollicular hemorrhages and trichomalacia are present (Figure 7.4a). Catagen hairs are greatly increased and are best seen in horizontal sections (Figures 7.4b,c).

Investigation and Diagnosis

A careful history must be taken in an understanding and non–confrontational manner. The clinical appearance is often diagnostic, but in some cases a scalp biopsy may be required. A psychiatric evaluation is sometimes necessary.

Differential Diagnosis

Other causes of patchy non-scarring alopecia such as alopecia areata, loose anagen syndrome, or tinea capitis must be excluded.

Treatment

Reassurance from the doctor and parental understanding and support will help the young child with a habit tic. Mentally retarded and older psychologically disturbed patients are much harder to treat, especially those with tonsure trichotillomania. Psychiatric care may help some of them, and antidepressive drugs or pimozide may be useful. ■

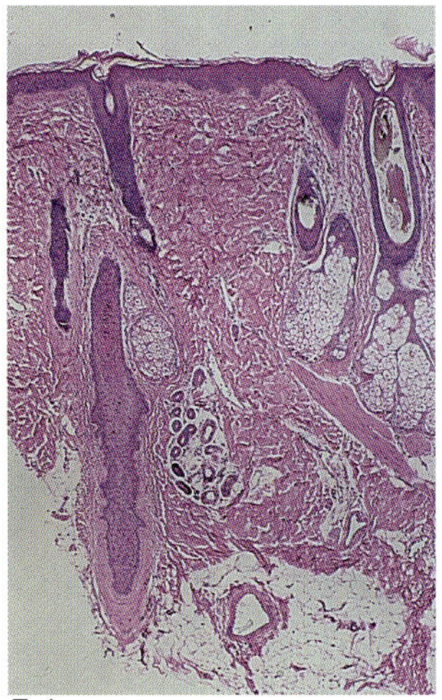

7.4a →

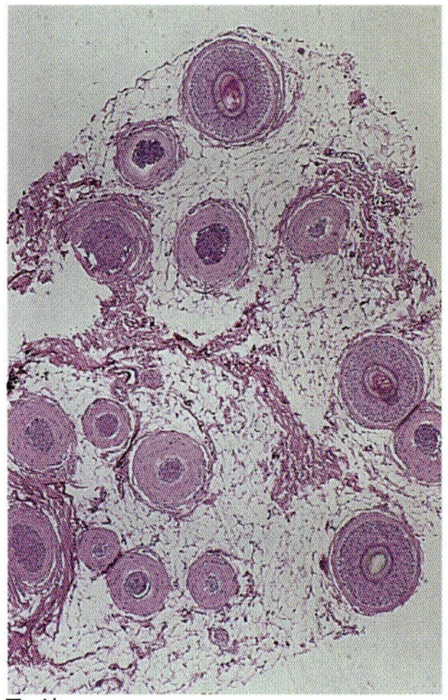

7.4b →

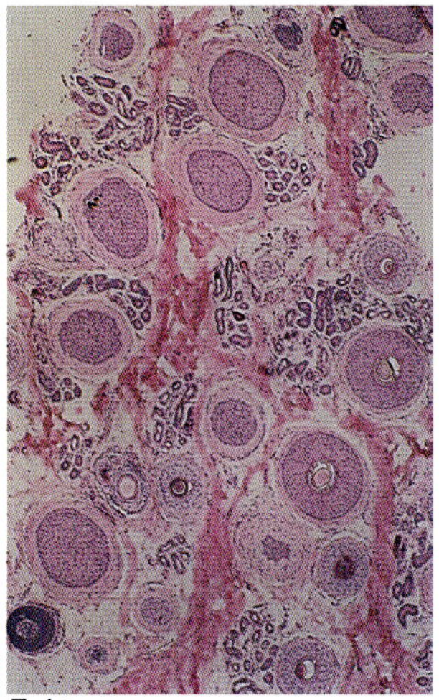

7.4c ■

7.4
Scalp biopsy: Histopathology of trichotillomania:

a. Vertical section: Trichomalacia is present in one follicular infundibulum and a catagen hair is visible in the lower dermis. There is a lack of inflammatory change. LM x 40.

b. Horizontal section: Subcutaneous level: Some catagen hairs are present here. LM x 40.

c. Horizontal section: Dermal level: Many catagen hairs are present and no inflammatory changes are seen. LM x 40. (*Reprinted with permission, Whiting, D.A., The Diagnosis of Alopecia, Current Concepts, Upjohn, 1990.*)

Suggested Reading

Dawber, R.: "Self–induced hair loss." *Semin Dermatol* 1985;4:53–57.

DeVillez, R.L.: "Infections, physical, and inflammatory causes of hair and scalp abnormalities." In: *Disorders of Hair Growth. Diagnosis and Treatment*, Olsen, E.A. (Ed.). New York: McGraw-Hill 1994:79–82.

Goldsmith, L.A., Baden, H.P.: "Mechanical properties of hair: Chemical modifications and pathological hairs." *J Invest Dermatol* 1971;56:200–204.

Hall-Smith, S.P.: "Familial trichotillomania." *Trans St. John's Hosp Derm Soc* 1966;52:135.

Jillson, O.F.: "Alopecia. II.Trichotillomania (trichotillohabitus)." *Cutis* 1983;31:383,386,389.

Lachapelle, J.M., Pierard, G.E.: "Traumatic alopecia in trichotillomania: a pathogenic interpretation of histologic lesions in the pilosebaceous unit." *J Cutan Pathol* 1977;4:51–67.

Mehregan, A.H.: "Trichotillomania: a clinicopathologic study." *Arch Dermatol* 1970;102:129–133.

Miescher, V.G., Schmiziger, P.: "Trichomalacie und trichotillomanie." *Dermatologica* 1957;114:199–203.

Muller, S.A.: "Trichotillomania." *Dermatol Clin* 1987;5:595–601.

Muller, S.A.: "Trichotillomania: A histopathologic study of sixty-six patients." *J Am Acad Dermatol* 1990;23:56–62.

Muller, S.A., Winkelmann, R.K.: "Trichotillomania: A clinicopathologic study of 24 cases." *Arch Dermatol* 1972;105:535–540.

Sanderson, K.V., Hall-Smith, P.: "Tonsure trichotillomania." *Br J Dermatol* 1970;82:343–350.

Steck, W.D.: "The clinical evaluation of pathologic hair loss with a diagnostic sign in trichotillomania." *Cutis* 1979;24:293–301.

Wilkin, J.K.: "Trichotillomania associated with alopecia areata." *Cutis* 1983;31:65– 66.

Alopecia Due to Other Causes of Traction and Trauma

Definition

Traction or traumatic alopecia results from various types of physical or chemical injury which may be acute or chronic.

Etiology

Traction alopecia can result from tight ponytails, cornrowing, braiding, backcombing, excessive brushing and combing and hair weaving. Other causes of physical trauma include the excessive application of heat, hot combing, and prolonged pressure on the scalp in the newborn or in ill, comatose or anesthetized patients. Vigorous scratching and pulling in seborrheic dermatitis, pediculosis capitis and psoriasis can cause alopecia, as can head rolling and banging, habit tics, neurotic excoriations, prurigo and lichen simplex. Chemical trauma results from excessive salt water bathing, frequent shampooing, and overexposure to setting lotions, permanent wave lotions and hair dyes.

Clinical Description

Alopecia involving scalp hair margins, provided alopecia areata and tinea capitis are excluded, generally results from chronic traction. This can be due to sustained traction from tight ponytails (Figures 8.1, 8.2, 8.3), braiding (Figure 8.4a), cornrowing, or forcible straightening of kinky hair. Patchy alopecia may result from brush rollers, hot combing, massaging and hair weaving (Figure 8.4b). Excessive brushing and backcombing can cause similar problems. Pressure alopecia is generally seen on the occipital or parietal areas from prolonged pressure on those areas in the immobile patient, who may be severly injured, very ill, comatose, or anesthetized (Figures 8.5a,b). Chemical alopecia from hair dyes, setting lotions and permanent waves can cause patches of broken off hairs (Figures 8.6a,b) and shampoos with cationic detergents can cause matted hair (Figure 8.6c). Habit tics, head rolling and banging, neurotic excoriations and prurigo are usually easy to diagnose clinically. Pruritic dermatoses such as seborrheic dermatitis, or pediculosis capitis with associated eczema, excoriations, lymphadenopathy, and possible nits, are easy to recognize as a rule.

(continued)

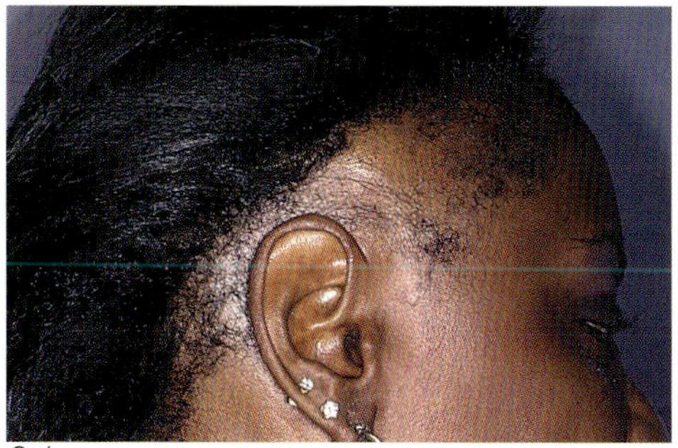
8.1

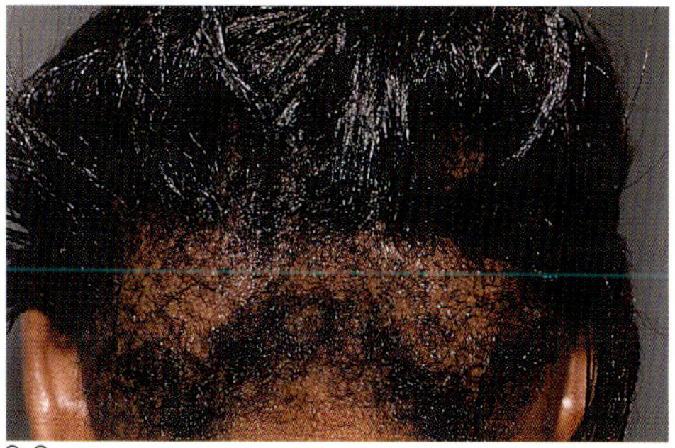
8.2

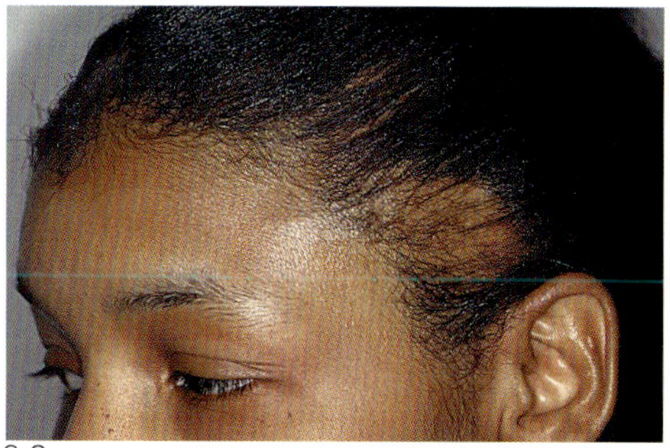
8.3

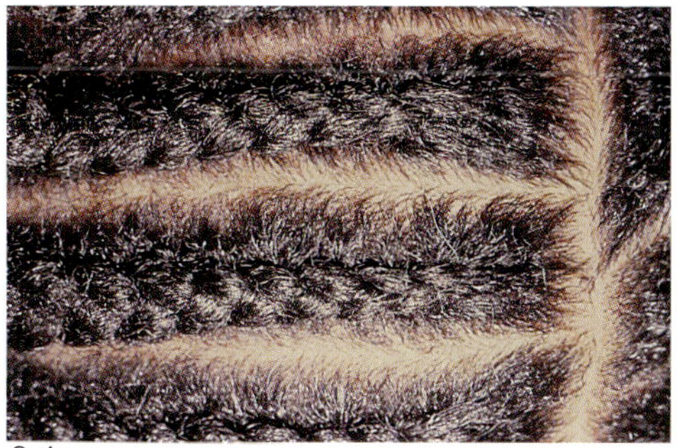
8.4a →

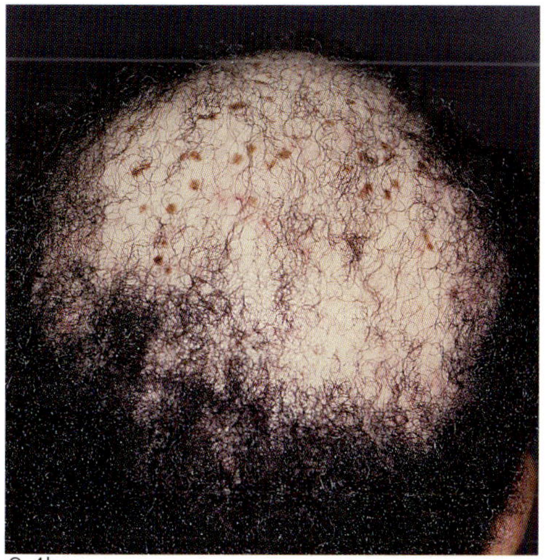
8.4b ■

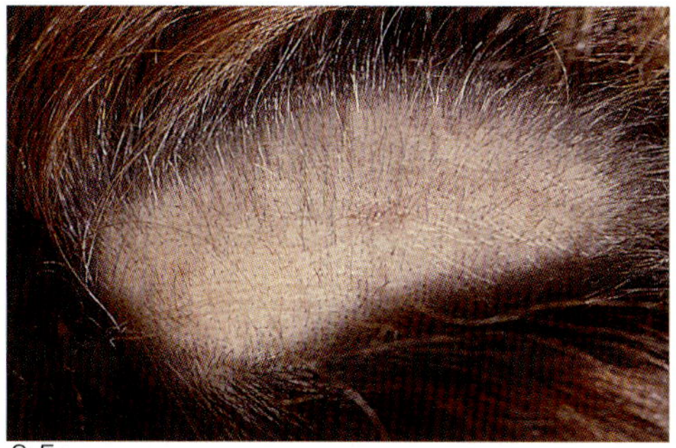
8.5a →

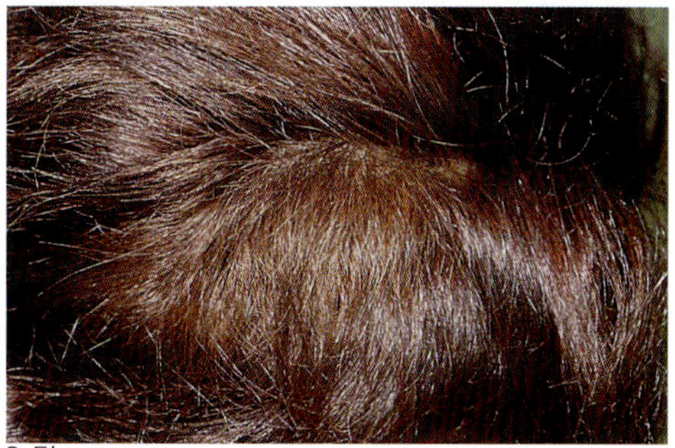
8.5b ■

8.1
Traction alopecia: Sustained traction from tight ponytail in childhood produced this band of alopecia at the frontotemporal hair margin.

8.2
Traction alopecia: Marginal alopecia over occiput from prolonged traction due to hair styling. *(Reprinted with permission, Whiting, D.A., The Diagnosis of Alopecia, Current Concepts, Upjohn, 1990.)*

8.3
Traction alopecia: Sustained traction from ponytail in childhood with constant application of greasy pomades has caused cicatricial, marginal alopecia in the left temporal area.

8.4
Traction alopecia:

a. Traction from tight braiding has led to linear areas of alopecia.

b. Persistent traction from a hair–weave has produced irregular alopecia around the margin of male pattern alopecia occurring in a patient with vitiligo.

8.5
Pressure alopecia:

a. Continuous pressure on patient's scalp during 8 hour cardiac bypass surgery led to rapid, patchy hair loss from area of pressure 10 days after operation.

b. Full regrowth of hair in patch of pressure alopecia 3 months later. *(Reprinted with permission, Whiting, D.A., The Diagnosis of Alopecia, Current Concepts, Upjohn, 1990.)*

Histopathology

Histopathology varies according to the cause. Chronic traction from hair weaves and other causes can produce a histopathological picture very similar to trichotillomania. There may be a lack of inflammation, but plugged follicles and melanin casts may be seen with an increased number of catagen and telogen hairs (Figures 8.7a,b). Marginal alopecia from traction and hot oil can show hair loss, fibrosis, and a deep perifolliculitis (Figures 8.8a,b,c).

Investigation and Diagnosis

A careful history and physical examination will clarify the diagnosis in most cases. Scalp biopsies are sometimes necessary.

Differential Diagnosis

Traumatic alopecia can be confused with alopecia areata, tinea capitis, secondary syphilis, cicatricial alopecia, and trichotillomania. Careful clinical evaluation will exclude most of these causes.

Treatment

Treatment depends on the cause. If necessary, cosmetic habits should be changed. Accidental causes of trauma should be identified and avoided where possible. ■

8.6
Chemical alopecia:

a. Alopecia due to hair breakage from prolonged application of permanent wave solution.

b. Chemical alopecia in contact dermatitis: Prolonged application of hair dye has caused contact dermatitis and alopecia from brittle hair.

c. Matted hair: Alopecia due to tangled hair caused by repeated shampoos containing a cationic detergent.

8.7
a,b. Scalp biopsy: Histopathology of traction alopecia due to hair–weave: Horizontal section: Lower dermis: Many catagen hairs are visible. There is no inflammatory change and no fibrosis. (a) LM x 40. (b) LM x 100.

8.8
Scalp biopsy: Histopathology of marginal traction alopecia:

a. Vertical section: Cicatricial alopecia – marked loss of terminal hairs is present and fibrosis is visible around one lower follicle in which a catagen hair is seen. LM x 40.

b. Horizontal section: Lower dermis: Cicatricial alopecia – only 3 follicular units are present and perifollicular fibrosis is seen. Catagen hair is visible. LM x 40.

c. Horizontal section: Upper dermis: Cicatricial alopecia – 3 follicular units are seen with follicles surrounded by fibrosis. LM x 40.

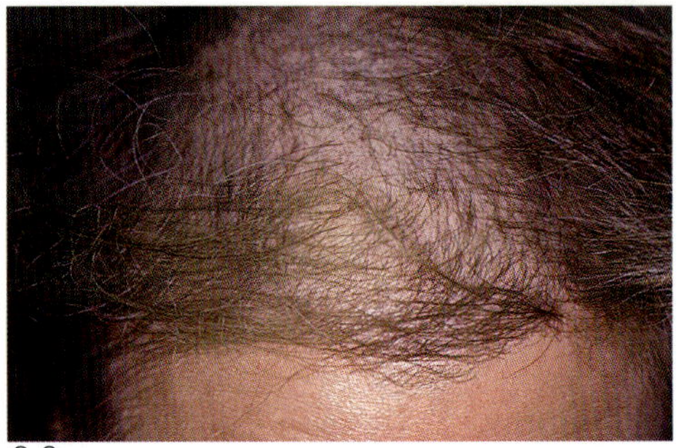

8.6a →

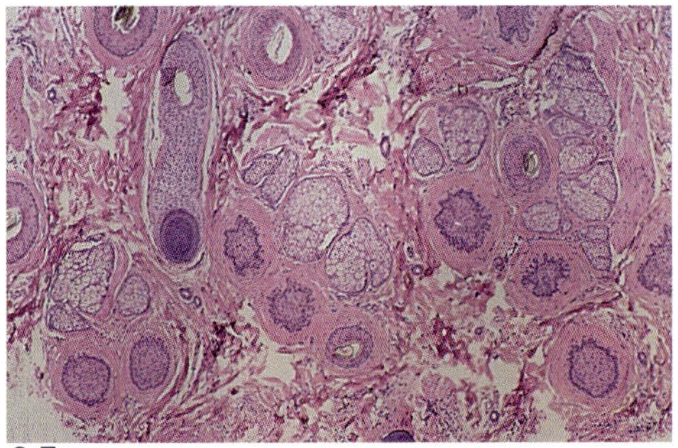

8.7a →

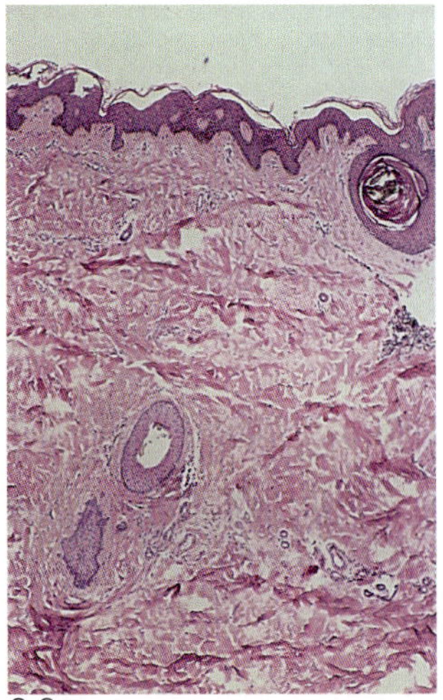

8.8a →

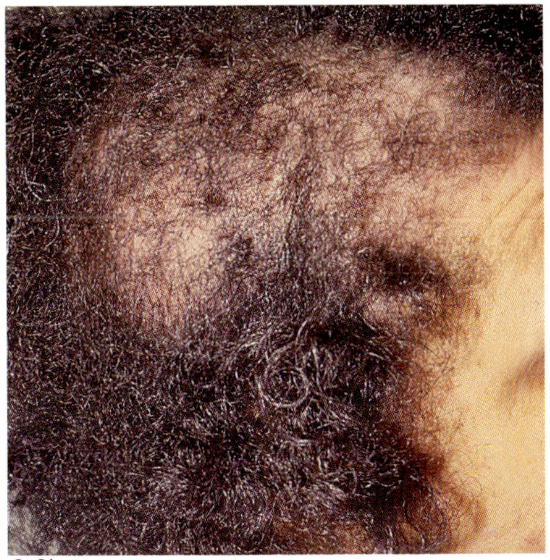

8.6b →

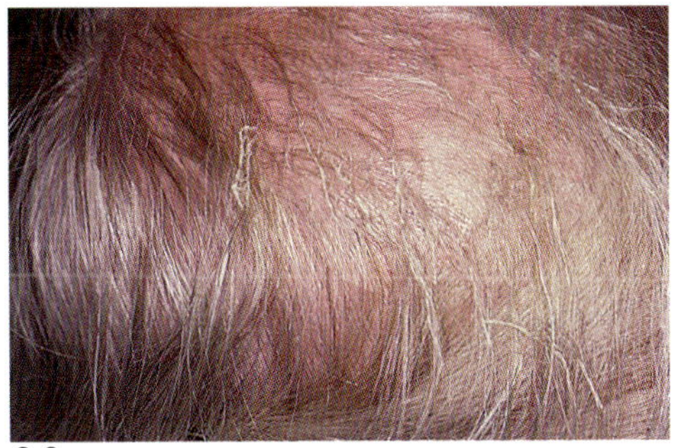

8.6c ■

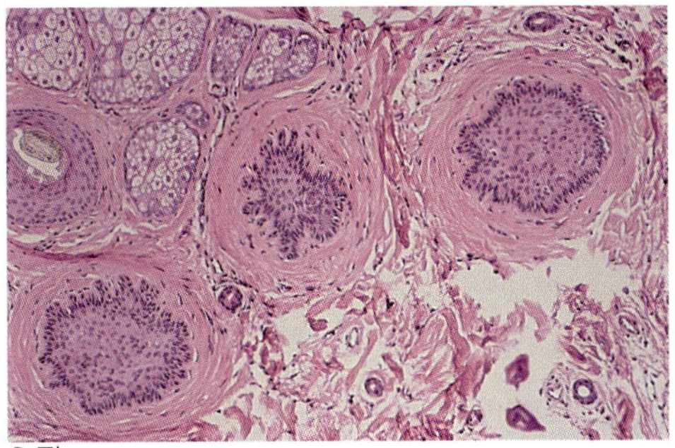

8.7b ■

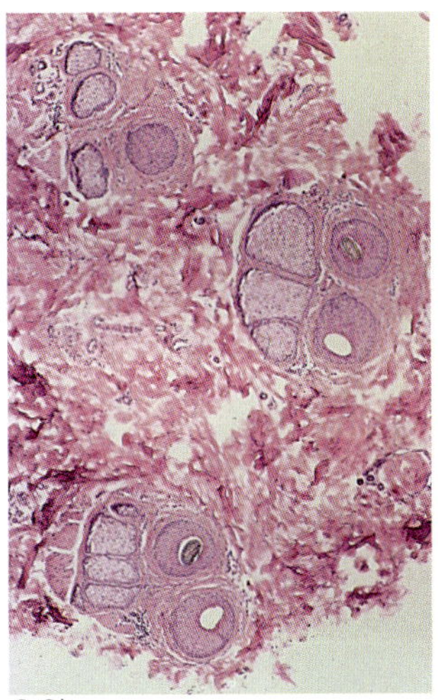

8.8b →

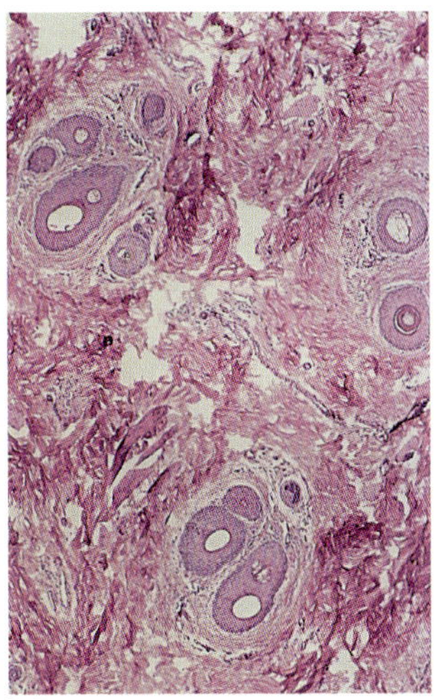

8.8c ■

Suggested Reading

Abel, R.R.: "Postoperative (pressure) alopecia." *Anesthesiology* 1964;25:869–871

Abel, R.R., Lewis, G.M.: "Postoperative (pressure) alopecia." *Arch Dermatol* 1960;81:34–42.

Aranoff, S.M., Levy, H.B., Tuchman, A.J., et al.: "Alopecia in meralgia paresthetica." *J Am Acad Dermatol* 1985;12:195–198

Berger, G.S., Peterson, B.: "Pressure alopecia after microsurgical anastomosis." *Am J Obstet Gynecol* (letter) 1978;704.

Bowers, R.E.: "Massage alopecia." *Br J Dermatol* 1950;62:262–264.

Bulengo-Ransby, S.M., Bergfeld, W.F.: "Chemical and traumatic alopecia from thioglycolate in a black woman: A case report with unusual clinical and histologic findings." *Cutis* 1992;49:99–103.

Corbett, J.F.: "Changing the color of hair." In *Principles of Cosmetics for the Dermatologist*. Frost, P., Horwitz, S.N. (Eds.). St. Louis: C. V. Mosby, 1982.

Corbett, J.F.: "Hair Dye Toxicity." In *Hair Research,* Orfanos, C.E., Montagna, W., Stuttgen, G. (Eds.). Berlin: Springer Verlag, 1981.

Earles, R.M.: "Surgical correction of traumatic alopecia marginalis or traction alopecia." *J Dermatol Surg Oncol* 1986;12:78.82.

Fischer, H., Caurdy, B.L.: "Scalp burns from a permanent wave product." *Clin Pediatr* 1990;29:53.

Gormley, T., Sokoll, M.D.: "Permanent alopecia from pressure of headstrap." *J Am Med Assoc* 1967;199:747–748.

Hjorth, N.: "Traumatic marginal alopecia. A special type – alopecia greenlandia." *Br J Dermatol* 1957;69:319–320

Lawson, N.W., Mills, N.L., Ochsner, J.L.: "Occipital alopecia following cardiopulmunary bypass." *J. Therac Cardiovasc Surg* 1976;71:342–347.

Lipnik, M.J.: "Traction alopecia from brush rollers." *Arch Dermatol* 1961;84:493– 495.

Lo Presti, P., Papa, C.M., Kligman, A.M.: "Hot comb alopecia." *Arch Dermatol* 1968;98:234–238.

Malhotra, Y.K., Kanwar, A.J.: "Tractional alopecia among Libyan women." (Letter) *Arch Dermatol* 1980;116:987.

Morgan, H.V.: "Traction alopecia." *Br Med J* 1960;ii:115–117.

Patel, K.D., Henschel, E.O.: "Postoperative alopecia." *Anaesthesia and Analgesia* 1980;59:311–313.

Perlstein, H.H.: "Traction alopecia due to hair weaving." *Cutis* 1969;5:440.

Rollins, T.G.: "Traction folliculitis with hair casts and alopecia." *Am J Dis Child* 1961;101:639–640.

Rudolf, R.I., Klein, A.W., Decherd, J.W.: "Corn-row alopecia." Arch *Dermatol* 1973;108:134.

Singh, G.: "Traction alopecia in Sikh boys." *Br J Dermatol* 1975;92:232–233.

Van Neste, D.: "Headgear induced traumatic alopecia during orthodontic treatment." In *Trends in Human Hair Growth and Alopecia Research.* Eds. Van Neste, D., Lachapelle, J.M., Antoine J.L. Dordrecht: Kluwer Academic Publishers, 1989:321– 324.

Wiles, J.C., Hansen, R.C.: "Postoperative (pressure) alopecia." *J Am Acad Dermatol* 1985;12:195–198.

Zuehlke, R.L., Bishara, S., Price, V.: "Pressure potentiated alopecia areata." *Am J Orthodont* 1981:437–438.

Alopecia Due to Infections and Infestations

Definition

Here the hair loss is related directly or indirectly to the destruction of the hair shaft or impairment of follicular function by microorganisms (dermatophyte, yeast, bacteria or virus) or to infestation by lice. Alopecia of this type will be considered by specific causative agent.

Fungal Infections

Dermatophytes:
Scalp ringworm results from an infection by any one of a number of fungal organisms known as dermatophytes. Dermatophytes are fungi which can colonize keratinized structures, namely stratum corneum, hair and nail. While often classified as anthropophilic, zoophilic or geophilic fungi by virtue of their source in man, animals, or soil, such classification is of little benefit in the diagnosis and treatment of tinea capitis. The manner of hair invasion, whether ectothrix, with spores occurring primarily on the outer surface of the hair shaft, or endothrix with spores filling the cortex of the hair shaft, is an organism-specific characteristic which is readily determined by examining affected hairs in a potassium hydroxide (KOH) preparation. While anthropophilic organisms generally induce less of an inflammatory response than organisms from other sources, under certain circumstances almost any clinical picture can be caused by any dermatophyte. The recognized clinical patterns include endothrix or black dot scalp ringworm, ectothrix scalp ringworm, kerion and favus.

Endothrix or black-dot scalp ringworm often presents as ill defined patches of partial alopecia, studded with black dots (Figures 9.1a,b). These black dots represent the retention of broken off, coiled hairs filled with spores. This is the most common form of tinea capitis in the USA today where such cases are almost always due to *Trichophyton tonsurans*; however, other endothrix organisms such as *T. violaceum*, *T. soudanense*, and *T. mentagrophytes* (Figure 9.2) can cause the same clinical picture. The lack of inflammation, as well as the diffuse pattern of involvement, frequently makes this form of ringworm a diagnostic challenge. Removal of one of the black dots from the scalp by fine forceps or the point of a sharp (No.11) scalpel blade, and examination of the specimen in potassium hydroxide (KOH) under the light microscope, results in the diagnostic finding of a large-spore endothrix infection (Figure 9.1b).

Ectothrix scalp ringworm presents as solitary or multiple rounded patches of alopecia with broken-off hairs and a variable amount of associated inflammation and scaling (Figure 9.3a). This form of ringworm is almost exclusively a prepubertal condition. In the past the anthropophilic organism *Microsporum audouini* was the most common cause, often occurring in epidemics within school populations. This organism gives a greenish fluorescence when examined under Wood's light. In recent years zoophilic organisms have become more frequent causes of ectothrix scalp ringworm in the USA, *M. canis* being the most common of these, often inducing a much more significant inflammatory response than *M. audouini*. KOH examination of a hair infected with *M. canis* shows a small spore ectothrix infection (Figure 9.3b). *M. gypseum* can also cause an inflammatory tinea capitis (Figure 9.4).

Kerions are persistent, raised, boggy masses in the scalp caused by a marked inflammatory response to the presence of a dermatophyte (Figure 9.5). Zoophilic organisms are the usual cause; however, occasionally anthropophilic organisms can result in such intensely inflammatory lesions. Kerion is the most likely cause of any boggy abscess of the scalp, associated with alopecia, in a prepubertal child. The intense inflammatory reaction results in early loss of infected hairs and it is often difficult to obtain a suitable specimen of hair for confirmation of the diagnosis by KOH preparation.

Favus presents as a distinctive clinical pattern. The cause is *T. schoenleinii*, usually contracted in early childhood from an infected parent. Early lesions are concave, keratinous cups enlarging from a hair follicle, pierced by a hair shaft and called scutula. These combine to form yellowish masses of crumbly material sometimes referred to as asbestos-like (Figures 9.6a,b). Cases of favus occur sporadically in many parts of the world but constitute a relatively rare and insignificant frac-

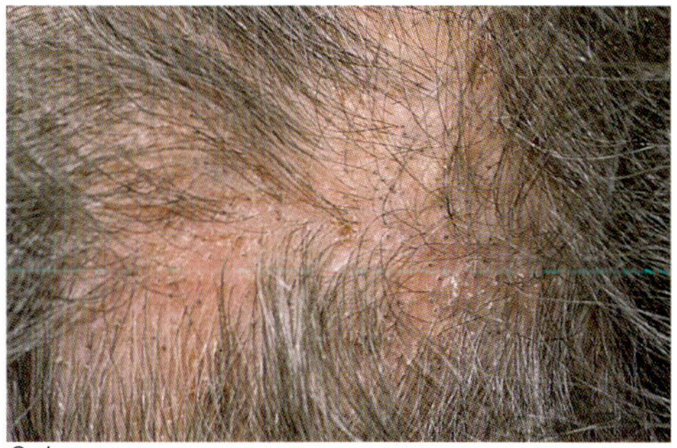
9.1a →

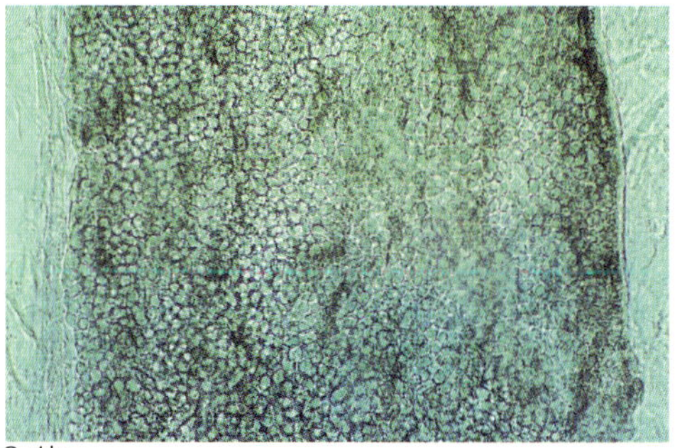
9.1b ■

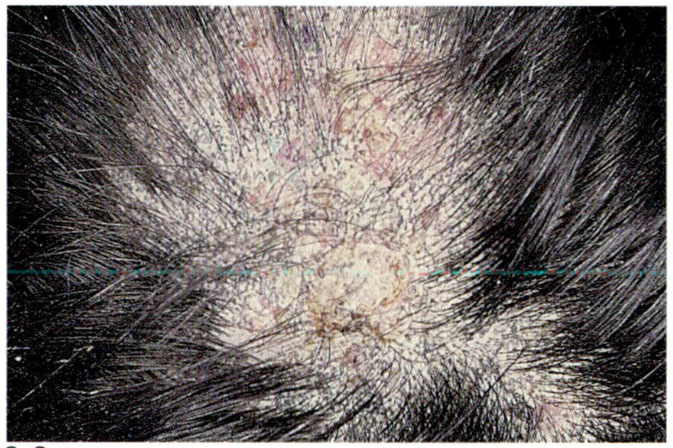
9.2

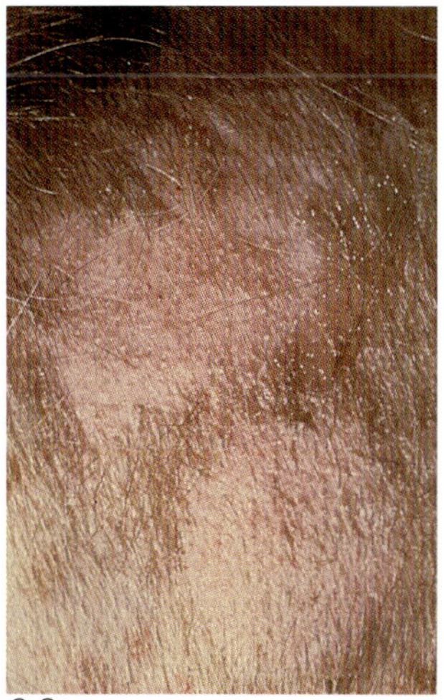
9.3a →

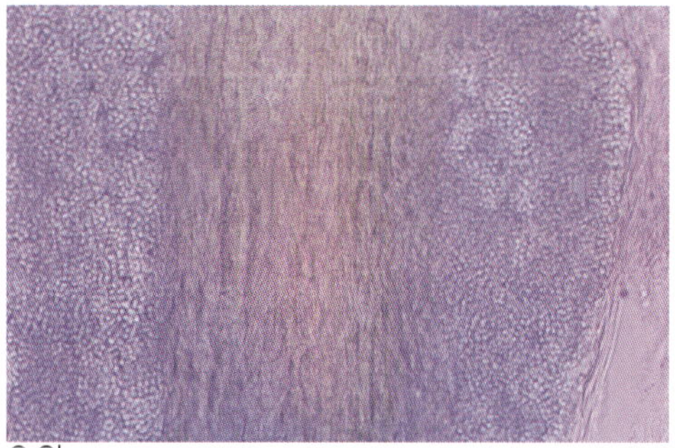
9.3b ■

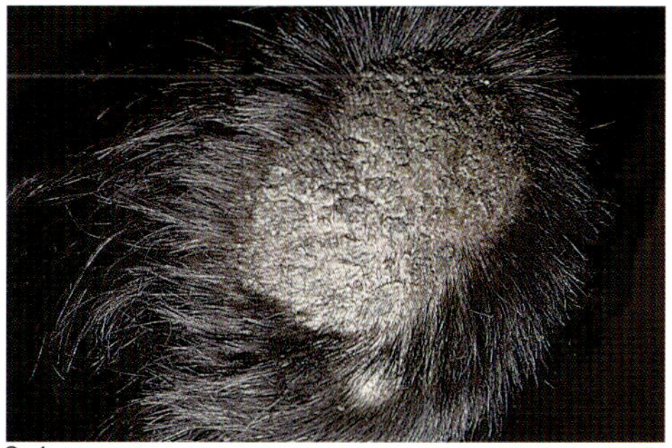
9.4

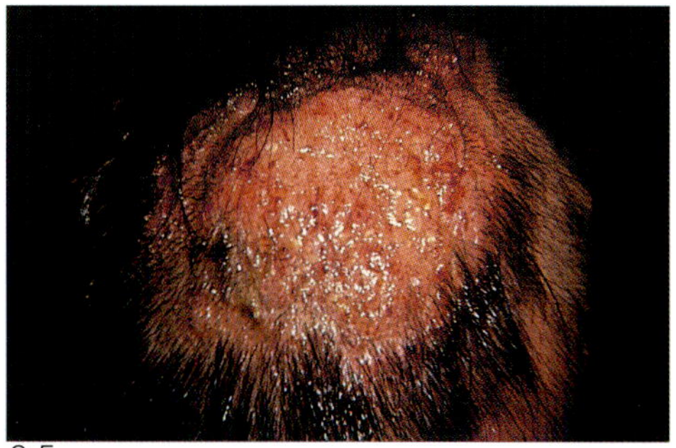
9.5

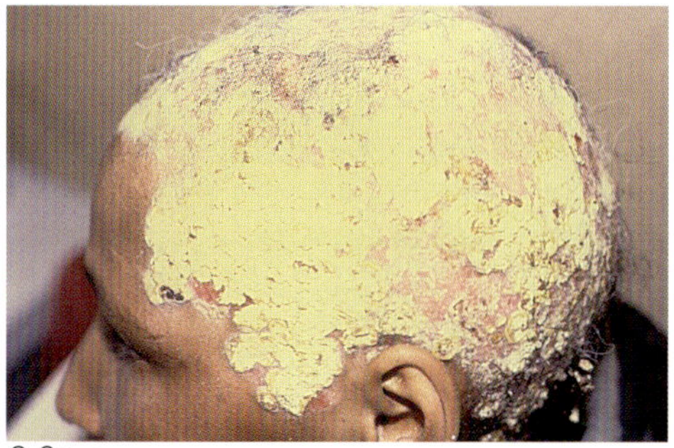
9.6a →

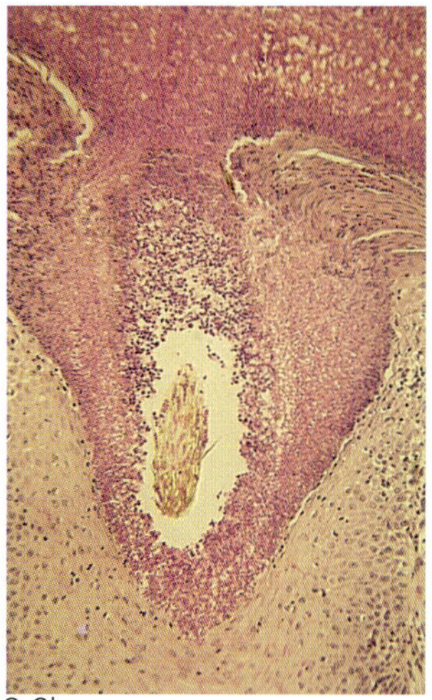
9.6b ■

9.1
Tinea capitis due to *Trichochophyton tonsurans:*

a. Black dots are clearly visible in an irregular area of alopecia of the scalp of an 80-year-old female. *(Reprinted with permission, Whiting, D.A., The Diagnosis of Alopecia, Current Concepts, Upjohn, 1990.)*

b. Potassium hydroxide preparation: Endothrix infection: The hair shaft is filled with large spores. LM x 400.

9.2
Tinea capitis due to *T. mentagrophytes:* Irregular patch of alopecia with crusting, inflammation and some black dots.

9.3
Tinea capitis: *Microsporum canis* infection:

a. Two annular patches of alopecia are seen containing traces of whitish stubble.

b. Potassium hydroxide preparation: Ectothrix infection: Many small fungal spores are present external to the hair shaft. LM x 400.

9.4
Tinea capitis due to *M. gypseum*. Large area of alopecia with severe crusting.

9.5
Kerion: Severe alopecia with granulation tissue, crusting and exudation.

9.6
Favus due to *T. schoenleinii:*

a. Extensive white crusting all over scalp due to confluence of scutula, leaving only a fringe of intact hair in the lower occipital and parietal areas. *(Courtesy of H. Francois Jordaan, M. Med.)*

b. Scalp biopsy: Histopathology of favus: Vertical section: Periodic Acid Shiff stain shows many spores in follicular infundibulum with overlying scutulum. LM x 100.

tion of all forms of tinea capitis. The alopecia from favus is usually permanent.

Treatment of all forms of tinea capitis requires systemic administration of an antifungal agent. Griseofulvin remains the treatment of choice; however, newer oral agents, including ketoconazole, fluconazole and itraconazole may be useful alternatives. The addition of systemic corticosteroids may minimize the scarring alopecia which often results from acutely inflamed kerions.

The diagnosis of scalp ringworm is usually confirmed by KOH examination of affected scalp hairs or by culture. On rare occasions histological examination of a scalp biopsy may reveal a previously undiagnosed fungal infection (Figures 9.7a,b).

Piedra:
While not generally responsible for significant alopecia, both black *(Piedraia hortai)* and white *(Trichosporon beigelii)* piedra are endemic in tropical environments. White piedra is now common in parts of the USA In both cases organisms invade the hair shaft and proliferate to form masses of hyphae in and around the hair shaft. In the case of black piedra the concretions are hard and dark, and in white piedra are soft, friable and nearly white. *T. beigelii* is believed to be more damaging to the hair shaft than *P. hortai* and may result in trichorrhexis nodosa and splitting.

For effective treatment, cut off all affected hairs and institute daily washing. Combination therapy with a topical imidazole compound such as 1% econazole nitrate, and oral ketoconazole, may be helpful.

Candidiasis:
Only chronic mucocutaneous candidiasis has the potential for causing alopecia. Chronic mucocutaneous candidiasis is represented by persistent candida infection of mouth, skin and nails from early childhood. Various immunological defects may be responsible; the scalp is not infrequently involved with hypertrophic, granulomatous plaques.
Oral antifungal agents such as ketoconazole, fluconazole and itraconazole are indicated in the treatment of chronic mucocutaneous candidiasis, often for prolonged periods.

Bacterial Infections

Trichomycosis Axillaris:
Trichomycosis axillaris is caused by *Corynebacterium tenuis*. Masses of bacteria form irregular nodules along the hair shaft of variable color, usually yellow, but in tropical climates occasionally red or black. This process is limited to axillary and occasionally pubic or scrotal hair.

The treatment is to cut off all affected hairs and wash the axillae regularly. Topical 1% clindamycin may be effective.

Folliculitis:
Furuncles, carbuncles, chronic folliculitis and perifolliculitis, acne necrotica (Figure 9.8), and erysipelas can result in alopecia. Treatment with suitable topical or systemic antibiotics may be required on a long-term basis.

Syphilis:
Hair loss associated with syphilis is seen during the secondary stage (Figures 9.9a,b,c,d) and is most commonly seen as a diffuse but patchy loss referred to as moth-eaten in appearance. Serological tests for syphilis should be performed in patients with diffuse loss where the diagnosis is in doubt. Severe alopecia can occur in congenital syphilis (Figure 9.10). Treatment with penicillin or other suitable antibiotics should result in hair regrowth within 4 to 6 weeks.

Leprosy:
While leprosy is known to cause the loss of the lateral third or even of all the eyebrow hair (Figure 9.11a), loss of scalp hair is unusual, but can sometimes occur in lepromatous, borderline, and tuberculoid leprosy (Figures 9.11b,c,d). Long-term treatment with a combination of drugs such as rifampin, dapsone, and clofazimine is necessary.

Viral Infections

Molluscum Contagiosum:
Molluscum contagiosum is commonly seen on the scalp in patients with acquired immunodeficiency syndrome where giant mollusca can cause patchy alopecia (Figure 9.12).

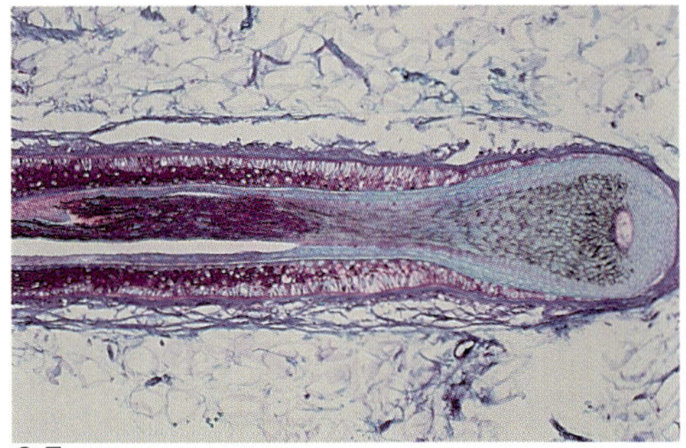

9.7a →

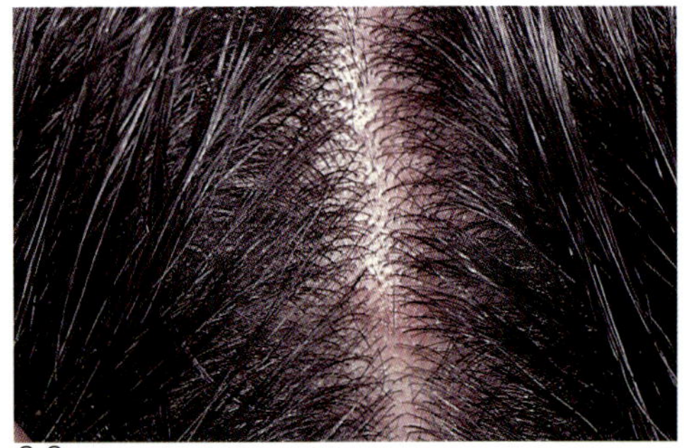

9.9a →

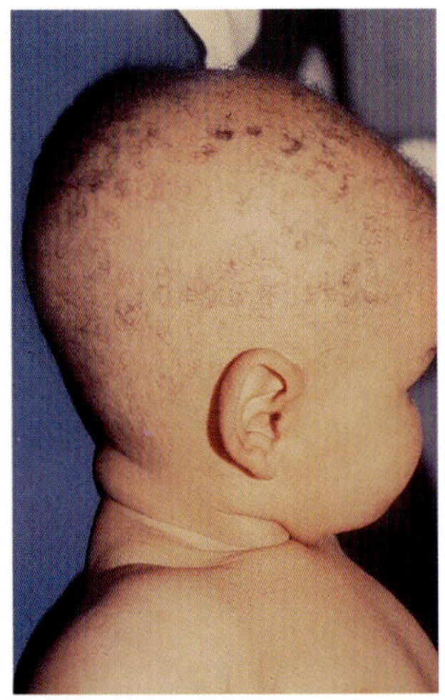

9.10

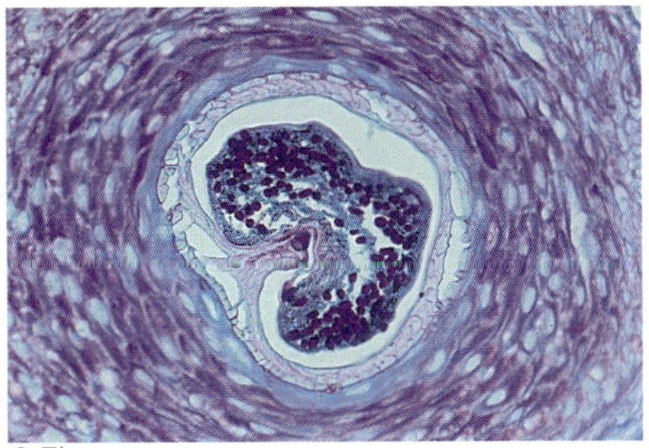

9.7b ■

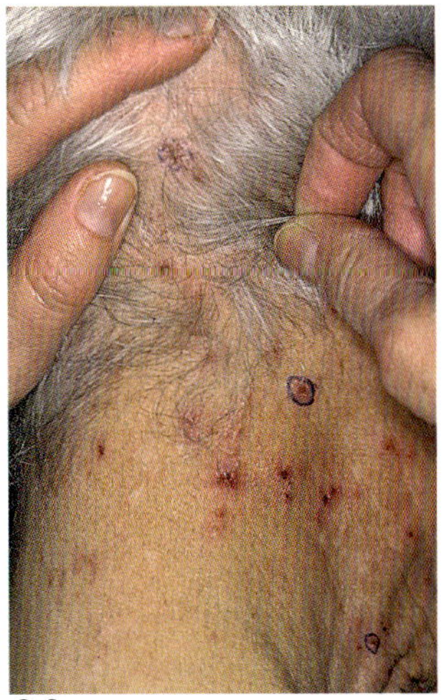

9.8

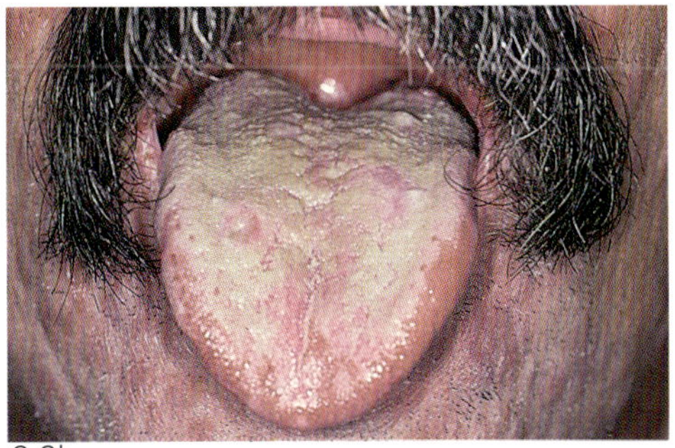

9.9b →

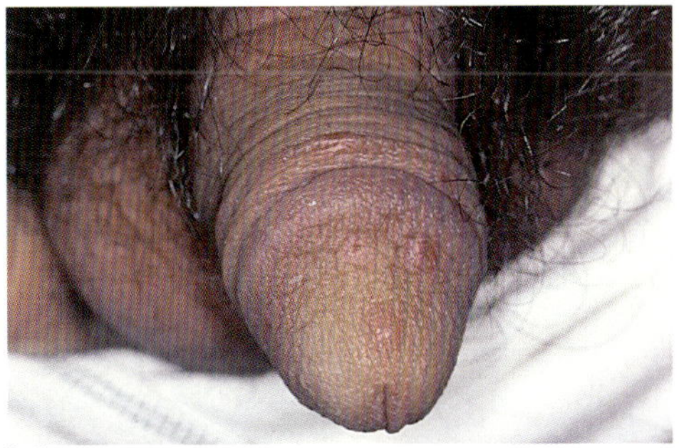

9.9c →

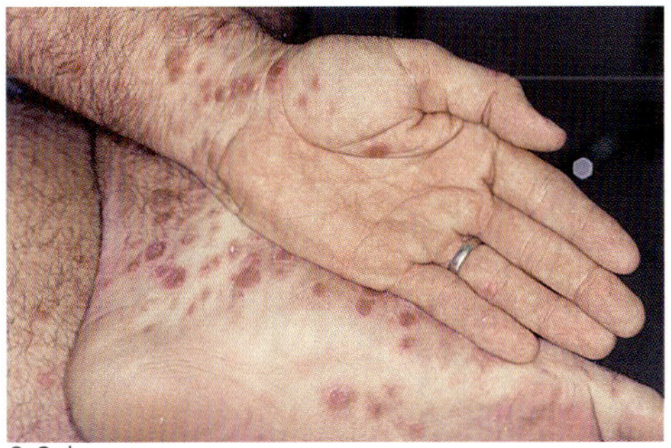

9.9d ■

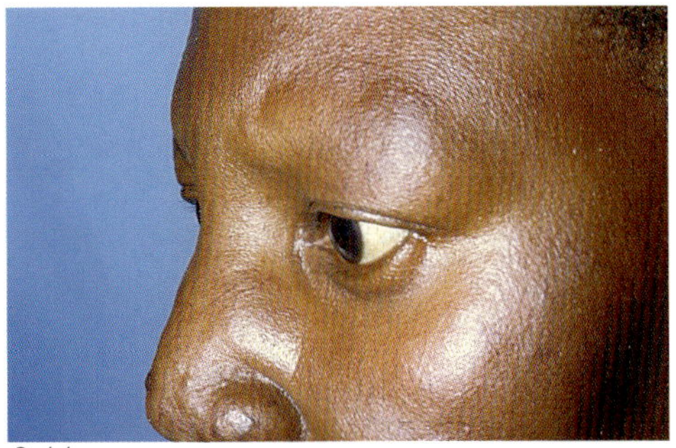

9.11a →

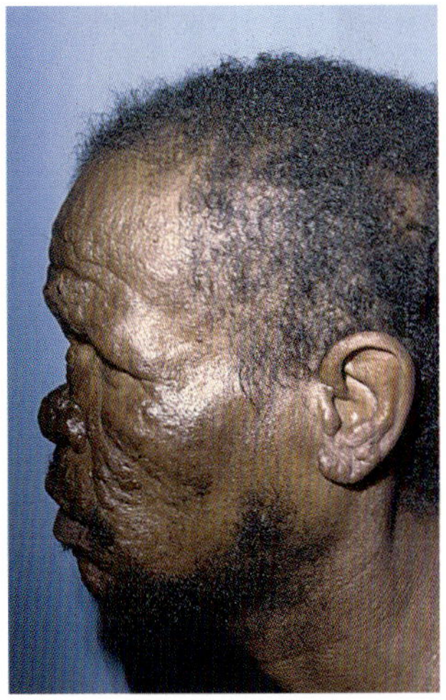

9.11b →

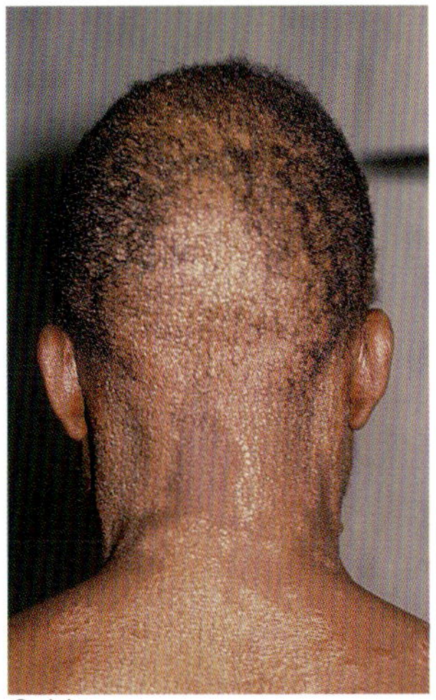

9.11c →

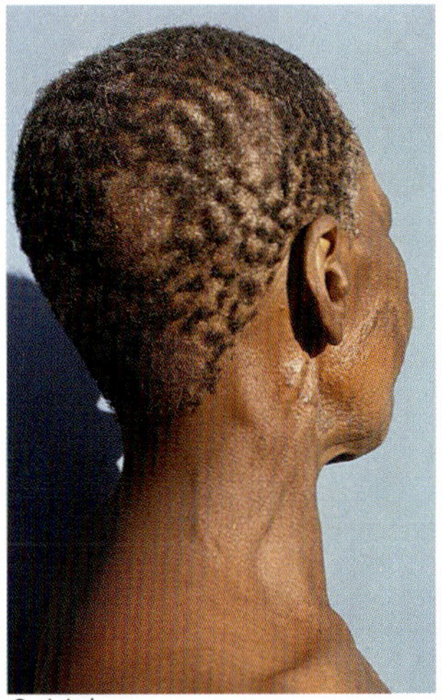

9.11d ■

9.7.
Scalp Biopsy: Histopathology of tinea capitis: Periodic Acid Shiff stain:

a. Vertical section: Fungal hyphae are seen in the cortex of the keratinizing hair. At the upper end of the hair a ridge of tissue from the internal root sheath is seen to penetrate the hair shaft. LM x 100.

b. Horizontal section: The hair shaft contains fungal spores and a grove in the hair shaft is penetrated by a ridge of internal root sheath. LM x 400.

9.8
Folliculitis: Acne miliaris necrotica with papulonecrotic lesions on the neck and extending into the occipital scalp.

9.9
Secondary syphilis:

a. Papules on scalp.

b. Mucous patches on tongue.

c. Papules on glans penis.

d. Maculopapular rash on palms and soles.

9.10
Baby with congenital syphilis showing crusting, dryness and scaling of scalp with severe alopecia. *(Courtesy of H. Francois Jordaan, M. Med.)*

9.11
Leprosy:

a. Lepromatous leprosy showing absence of eyebrows and eyelashes but presence of scalp hair. *(Courtesy of E.J. Schulz, M.Med.)*

b. Lepromatous leprosy with patchy alopecia of scalp and leonine facies. *(Courtesy of E.J. Schulz, M.Med.)*

c. Borderline leprosy showing patchy alopecia of scalp. *(Courtesy of H. Francois Jordaan, M. Med.)*

d. Tuberculoid leprosy showing patchy alopecia of scalp and thickened nerves in neck. *(Courtesy of E.J. Schulz, M.Med.)*

Methods of removal of individual lesions include cryosurgery, cauterization, and curettage.

Herpes Zoster:
Herpes zoster can lead to alopecia in a unilateral pattern when the ophthalmic division of either trigeminal nerve is involved. The associated pain and vesiculation usually point to the diagnosis, although histological examination of a scalp biopsy may be needed (Figures 9.13a,b). Any associated alopecia is generally transient unless significant scarring occurs. Early treatment with high doses of acyclovir is currently recommended.

Infestations

Pediculosis:
Head lice *(Pediculus humanus capitis)* are found throughout the world and are readily transmitted. Most commonly pre-school and school-aged children are infested; however, no age is exempt. Pruritus is a constant feature of infestation and is believed to be aggravated by a hypersensitivity to louse saliva. The developing and adult lice inject saliva in the process of feeding on human blood. The infestation and feeding occurs most densely on the occipital scalp, and excoriations, secondary infection, and cervical adenitis are frequently noted. The presence of egg cases, or nits, attached to the hair shaft are diagnostic (Figures 9.14a,b). These ovoid bodies are so firmly cemented to the hair shaft that they cannot be moved along it. The treatment of choice is 1% permethrin creme rinse; a suitable alternative is 1% lindane shampoo.

Insect Bites:
Insect bites, particularly tick bites, may result in an inflammatory papule which in turn may leave a small area of alopecia. In the case of the tick it is believed that a salivary anticoagulant is responsible for the alopecia. The tick bite may result in a patch of alopecia up to 4 cm in diameter which can resemble alopecia areata. However, in tick bite alopecia a central crust or punctum will generally be noted (Figure 9.15), and the hair usually regrows promptly. ■

9.12
Molluscum contagiosum: Giant molluscum on scalp in AIDS patient.

9.13
a,b. Scalp biopsy: Histopathology of herpes zoster: Vertical section: The follicular infundibulum and mid follicle are affected by the herpes zoster virus. Ballooning degeneration, reticular degeneration, intranuclear viral inclusions, and necrotic changes are seen. LM x 100.

9.14
Pediculosis capitis:

a. Many nits are seen attached to free ends of scalp hairs.*(Reprinted with permission, Whiting, D.A., Hair shaft defects, in Disorders of Hair Growth: Diagnosis and Treatment, Olsen, E.A. [Ed] McGraw-Hill, 1994.)*

b. Microscopic examination: A nit is seen attached to hair shaft capped by an intact operculum and containing a developing louse. LM x 100.

9.15
Tick bite alopecia: Central tick bite surrounded by area of alopecia caused by anticoagulants in tick saliva.

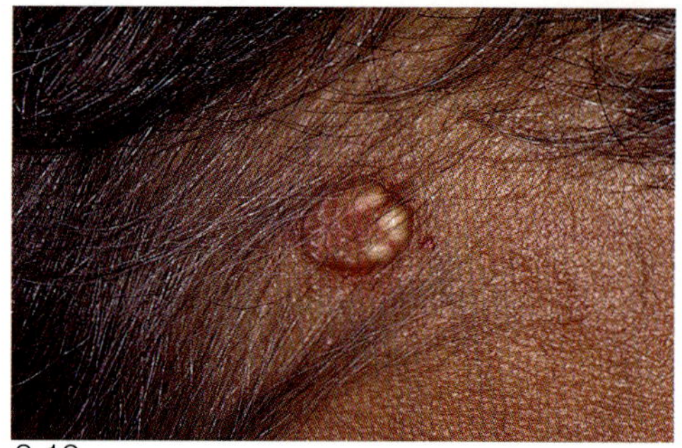

9.12

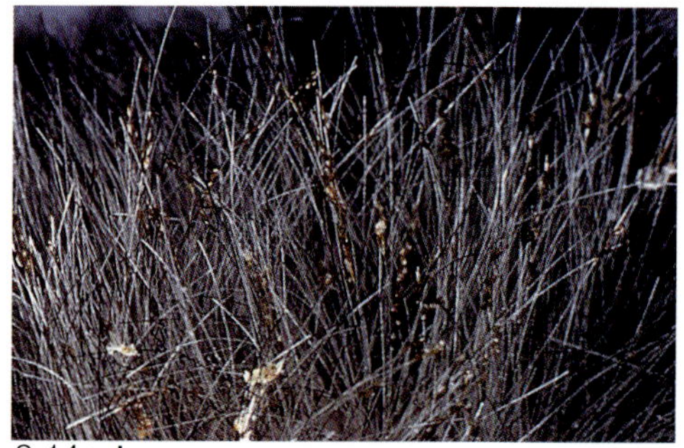

9.14a ↓

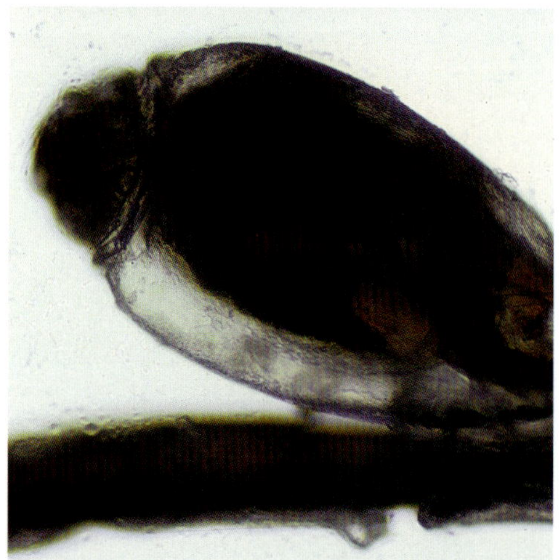

9.14b ■

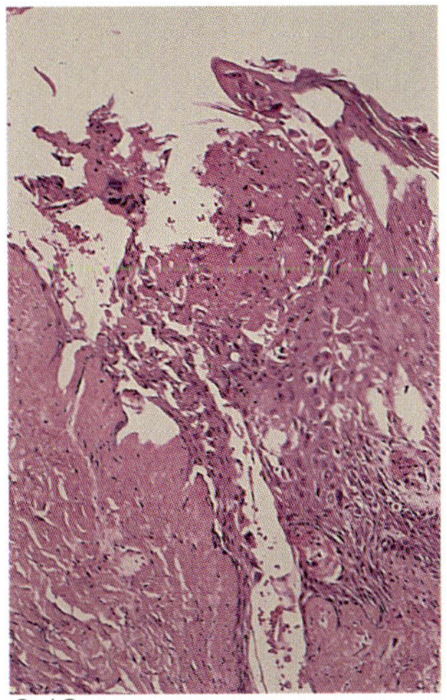

9.13a ↓

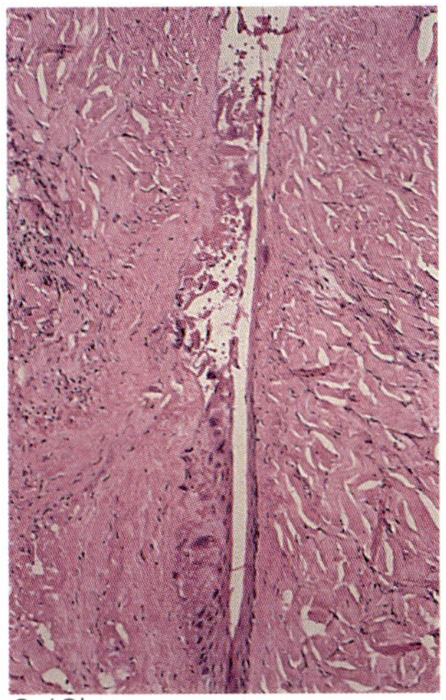

9.13b ■

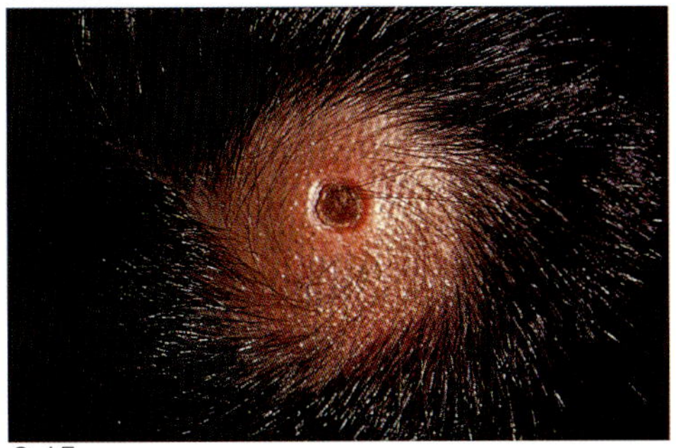

9.15

Recommended Reading

Amer, M.A., Taha, M., Diab, N.A., et al.: "Ultrastructure of *Trichophyton violaceum*." *Int J Dermatol* 1993;32:97–99.

Barlow, D., Saxe, N.: "Tinea capitis in adults." *Int J Dermatol* 1988;27:388–390.

Bronson, D.M., Desai, D.R., Barsky, S.: "An epidemic of infection with *Trichophyton tonsurans* revealed in a 20-year survey of fungal infection in Chicago." *J Am Acad Dermatol* 1983;8:322–330.

DeVillez, R.L.: "Infections, physical, and inflammatory causes of hair and scalp abnormalities." In: *Disorders of Hair Growth. Diagnosis and Treatment,* Olsen, E.A. (Ed.). New York: McGraw-Hill 1994:71–79.

Ellner, K.M., McBride, M.E., Kalter, D.C., et al.: "White piedra: evidence for a synergistic infection." *Br J Dermatol* 1990;123:355–363.

Fogel, E.K., Jepsen, L.V.: "Hair loss following kerion celci: a follow-up examination." *Mykosen.* 1984;27:411–414.

Freeman, R.G., McBride, M.E., Knox, J.M.: "Pathogenesis of trichomycosis axillaris." *Arch Dermatol* 1969;100:90–95.

Hauser, F.V., Rothman, S.: "Monilial granuloma: Report of a case and review of the literature." *Arch Dermatol Syphilol* 1950;61:297–310.

Kalter, D.C., Tschen, J.A., Cernoch, P.L., et al.: "Genital white piedra: epidemiology, microbiology and therapy." *J Am Acad Dermatol* 1986;14:982–993.

Kligman, A.M.: "The pathogenesis of tinea capitis due to *Microsporum audouini* and *Microsporum canis*." *J Invest Dermatol* 1952;18:231–246.

Kligman, A.M.: "Tinea capitis due to *M. audouini* and *M. canis*." *Arch Dermatol* 1955;71:313–357.

Lee, J. Y-Y., Hsu, M-L.: "Alopecia syphilitica, a simulator of alopecia areata: histopathology and differential diagnosis." *J Cutan Pathol* 1991;18: 87–92.

Lee, J. Y-Y., Hsu, M-L.: "Pathogenesis of hair infection and black dots in tinea capitis caused by *Trichophyton violaceum:* a histopathological study." *J Cutan Pathol* 1992;19:54–58.

Meinking, T.L., Taplin, D., Kalter, D.C., et al.: "Comparative efficacy of treatments for pediculosis capitis infestations." *Arch Dermatol* 1986;122:267–271.

Okuda, C., Ito, M., Sato, Y.: "Fungus invasion into human hair tissue in black dot ringworm: Light and electroscopic study." *J Invest Dermatol* 1988;90:729–733.

Orfanos, C.E., Schloesser, E., Mahrle, G.: "Hair destroying growth of *Corynebacterium tenuis* in the so-called trichomycosis axillaris." *Br J Dermatol* 1968;80:509–513.

Roberts, S.O.B., Mackenzie, D.W.R.: "Tinea capitis." In Rook, A., Wilkinson, D.S., Ebling, F.J.G., (Eds.) *Textbook of Dermatology,* (3rd ed.) Oxford: Blackwell Scientific Publications, 1979:793–798. (vol 1).

Rook, A., Dawber, R.: *Diseases of the Hair and Scalp. (2nd ed.)* Oxford: Blackwell Scientific Publications, 1991:396–457.

Rudolph, A.H.: "The diagnosis and treatment of tinea capitis due to *Trichophyton tonsurans*." *Int J Dermatol* 1985;24:426–431.

Sperling, L.C.: "Inflammatory tinea capitis (kerion) mimicking dissecting cellulitis. Occurrence in two adolescents." *Int J Dermatol* 1991;30:190–192.

Alopecia Due to Hair Shaft Abnormalities

Definition

The four major categories of structural abnormalities of the hair shaft comprise fractures (Figure 10.1), irregularities (Figures 10.2a,b), coiling and twisting (Figure 10.3), and extraneous matter (Figure 10.4) affecting the hair shaft.

Etiology

Hair shaft abnormalities can be inherited or acquired and may indicate underlying disease. Shaft abnormalities can occur in association with other defects in many congenital syndromes, particularly the ectodermal dysplasias. Physical and chemical trauma are important in the etiology of many hair shaft defects, both in normal or in fragile hair.

Clinical Description

Hair shaft abnormalities are classified in Table 10.1.

The abnormalities associated with structural weakness of the hair shaft, indicated with an asterisk, can give rise to hair breakage and loss. In these cases the distal hair shafts break off in fragments on gentle pulling, the so-called feathering technique. The extent of the abnormality will depend on the cause. Many of the inherited abnormalities are fairly diffuse. Abnormalities due to local trauma such as trichotillomania are more likely to be patchy.

Weathering: Weathering is the wear and tear that affects the free end of both normal and abnormal hairs. It is caused by a variety of physical and chemical factors such as excessive hair styling, washing, friction, sun, wind, and swimming. Cuticular cell margins erode at the free end of the hair exposing the underlying cortical fibers which fray. Split ends result.

When evaluating hair shaft abnormalities, examine the proximal 1 to 2 cm of a hair shaft adjacent to the scalp to exclude the effects of weathering. Remember that hair shaft abnormalities need to be found in different areas of the scalp since many hair shaft abnormalities can occur sporadically in normal hair with exceptions such as pili annulati, pili bifurcati and monilethrix. It is important to recognize normal variations of the hair cycle before diagnosing abnormalities.

Fractures of the Hair Shaft

Trichorrhexis Nodosa: Trichorrhexis nodosa is initiated by a loss of cuticular cells in one or more areas of the hair shaft. The exposed cortical fibers separate and fray producing a nodular swelling which resembles two paint brushes thrust into one another. With complete breakage the typical expanded fracture is seen. Clinically, the nodes appear as pale specks fixed to the hair shaft and may affect the proximal or the distal hairs (Figures 10.5a,b). The

10.1
Fractures of the hair shaft: Normal hair: Transverse fractures–trichorrhexis nodosa, trichoschisis, trichoclasis, trichorrhexis invaginata. Oblique fracture – tapered fracture. Longitudinal fracture–trichoptilosis.

10.2
a. Irregularities of the hair shaft: Longitudinal ridging and grooving, uncombable hair, loose anagen syndrome, pili bifurcati and pili annulati.

10.1

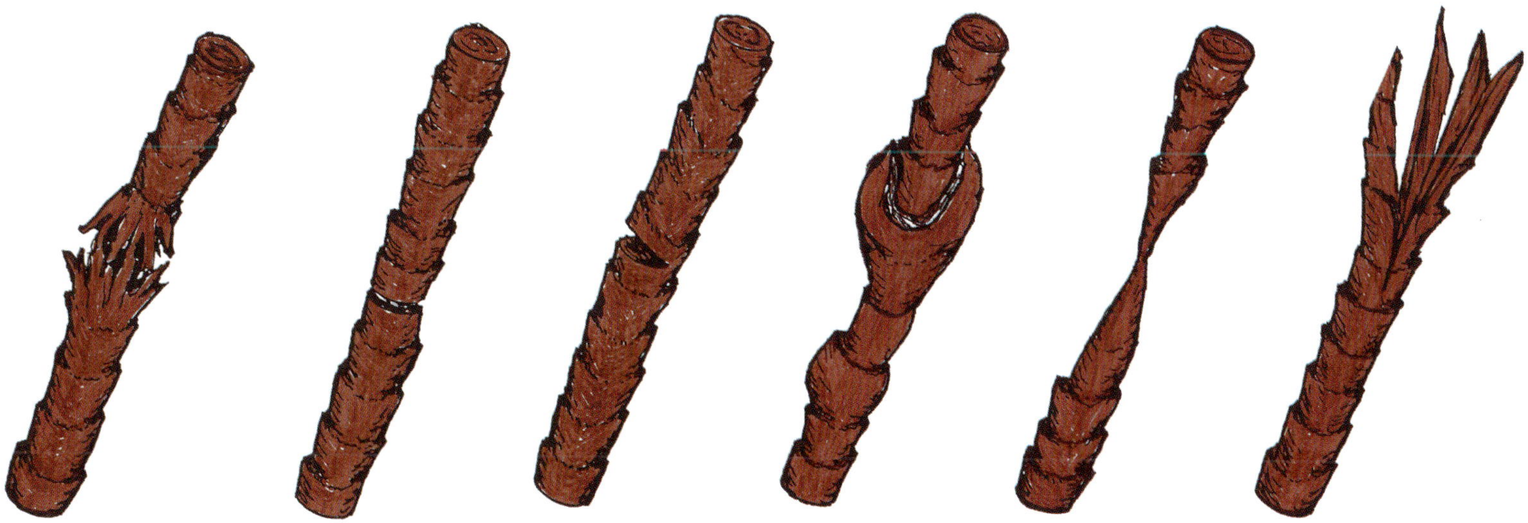

Trichorrhexis nodosa — Trichoschisis — Trichoclasis — Trichorrhexis invaginata — Tapered fracture — Trichoptilosis

10.2a

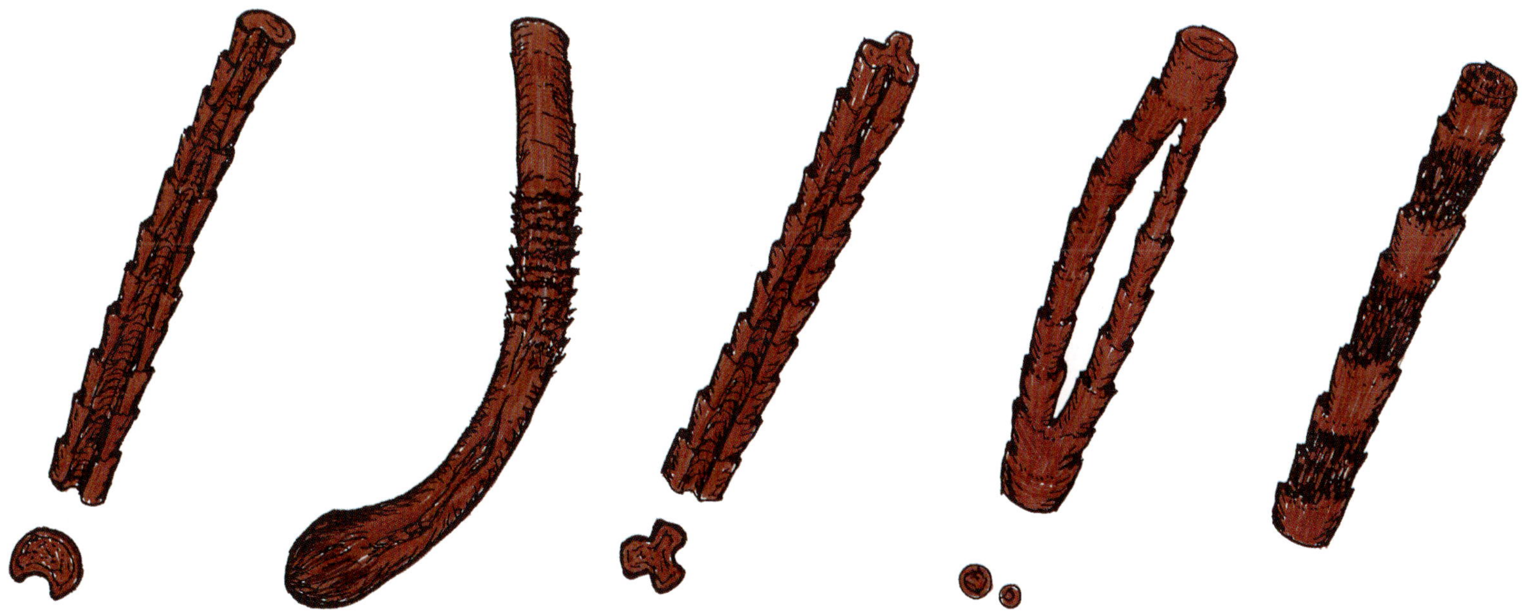

Longitudinal ridging and grooving — Loose anagen syndrome — Uncombable hair Pili trianguli — Pili bifurcati — Pili annulati

10.2
b. Irregularities of the hair shaft; Monilethrix, pseudomonilethrix, tapered hair, bayonet hair and bubble hair.

10.3
Coiling and twisting of the hair shaft: Pili torti, corkscrew hair, woolly hair, and trichonodosis and circle hairs.

10.4
Extraneous matter on the hair shaft: Tinea capitis, trichomycosis axillaris or piedra, pediculosis capitis and peripilar cast.

10.2b

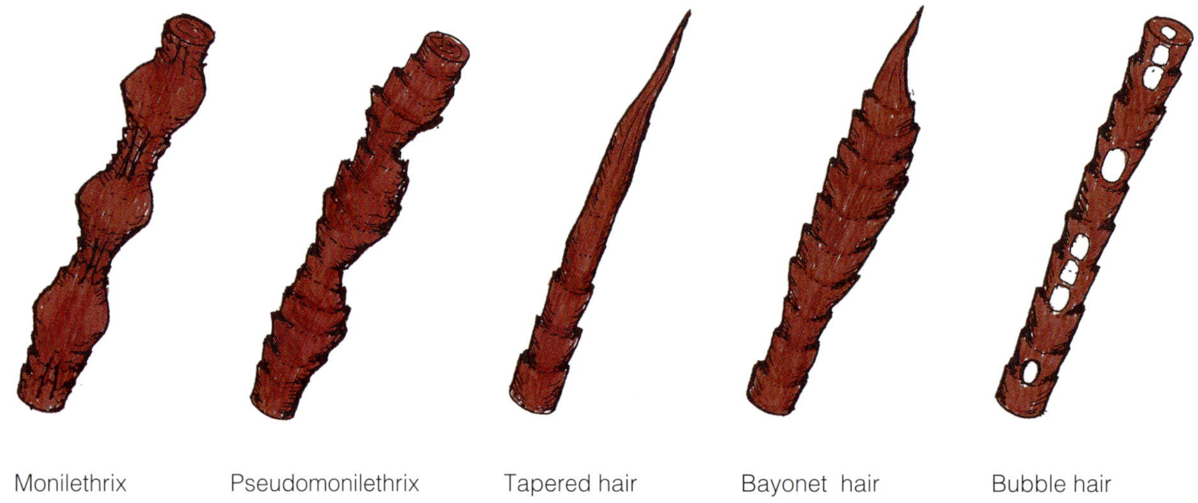

10.3

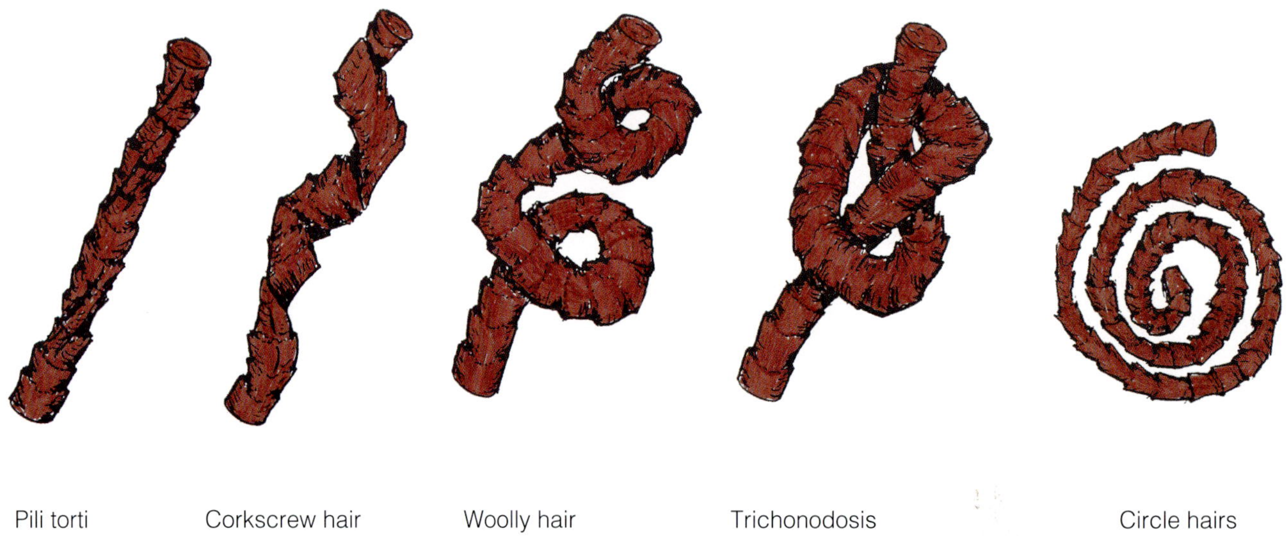

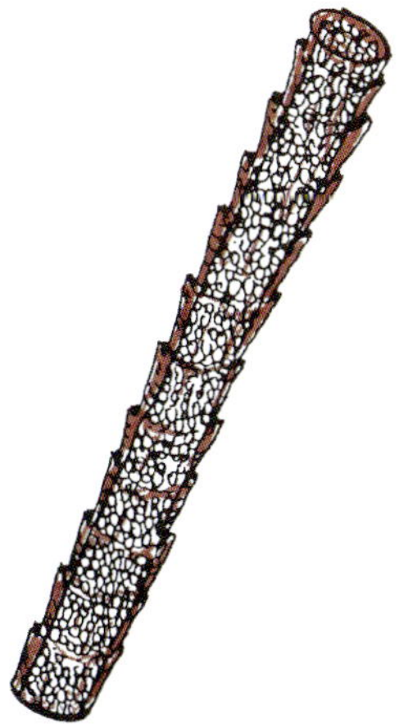

Tinea capitis

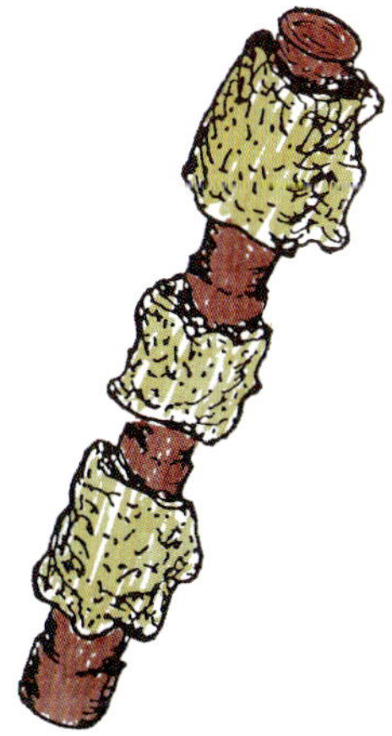

Trichomycosis axillaris
or piedra

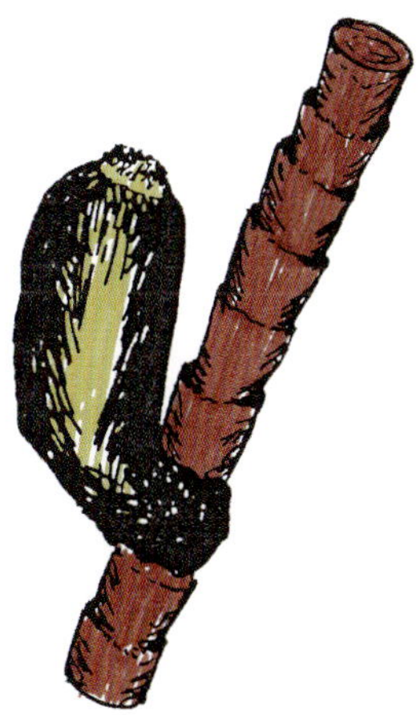

Pediculosis capitis

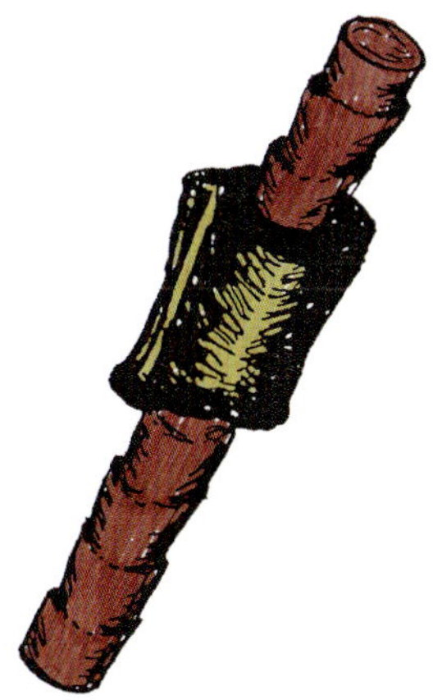

Peripilar cast

Table 10.1 Classification of hair–shaft abnormalities*

Fractures of the hair shaft	Transverse	**Trichorrhexis nodosa **Trichoschisis Trichoclasis **Trichorrhexis invaginata
	Oblique	**Tapered fracture
	Longitudinal	Trichoptilosis
Irregularities of the hair shaft		Longitudinal ridging and grooving, including loose anagen syndrome Uncombable hair or pili trianguli et canaliculi or spun glass hair, including straight hair nevus Pili bifurcati and pili multigemini, including trichostasis spinulosa Pili annulati Pseudopili annulati **Monilethrix **Pseudomonilethrix **Tapered hairs, including Pohl–Pinkus mark, bayonet hairs, tapered newly growing anagen hairs, and trichomalacia Bubble hairs **Intermittent hair–follicle dystrophy
Hair–shaft coiling and twisting		**Pili torti, including corkscrew hair and Menkes' syndrome Woolly hair, including acquired progressive kinking, acquired nonprogressive kinking, and whisker hair Trichonodosis (knotted hair) Circle hairs
Extraneous matter on the hair shaft	Fungi	Tinea capitis Piedra
	Bacteria	Trichomycosis axillaris
	Pediculosis	Nits
	Peripilar casts	Pseudonits
	Deposits	Lacquer, paint, glue

*After Whiting, D.A.: Structural abnormalities of the hair shaft. J Am Acad Dermatol 1987;16:1–25.
**Associated with hair fragility

basic cause of trichorrhexis nodosa is trauma and a contributory factor is inherent weakness of the hair shaft. Excessive weathering, backcombing, stressed hair styles, head rolling and banging, habit tics, trichotillomania, scratching, perming and dyeing of hair can cause trichorrhexis nodosa. It is aggravated by brittle hair such as that seen in pili torti, monilethrix, pseudomonilethrix, trichorrhexis invaginata, trichothiodystrophy, argininosuccinic aciduria, citrullinemia, and Menkes' disease. Trichorrhexis nodosa may be congenital or acquired. Congenital trichorrhexis nodosa may occur as an isolated entity or may occur with abnormalities such as argininosuccinic aciduria, citrullinemia, Menkes' disease, or trichothiodystrophy. Acquired proximal trichorrhexis nodosa is common in blacks and due to excessive hair straightening or other forms of hair styling. Acquired distal trichorrhexis nodosa occurs in whites or Orientals and is caused by excessive styling and brushing.

Trichoschisis: Trichoschisis is a clean transverse fracture across the hair shaft associated with a localized absence of cuticle cells. It results from trauma and is usually seen in the congenitally brittle hair of trichothiodystrophy, with a sulfur content 50% lower than normal. The hair shaft is often ribbonlike, with flattening and folding. Most fractures show the clean breaks of trichoschisis but others show the expanded appearance of trichorrhexis nodosa. Alternating bright and dark bands are seen in the hair shaft under polarized light (Figures 10.6a,b). The brittle hair of trichothiodystrophy may be associated with intellectual impairment, decreased fertility, short stature, ichthyosis, photosensitivity, and other abnormalities. Severe alopecia occurs in scalp, eyebrows and eyelashes. Hair is dry and coarse and it breaks off near the skin surface.

Trichoclasis: Trichoclasis is the common "greenstick" fracture in which a transverse fracture of the shaft is splinted in part by an intact cuticle. It is usually sporadic and is caused by physical and chemical trauma.

Trichorrhexis invaginata: Trichorrhexis invaginata is a nodular fracture of the hair shaft in which a ball and socket joint is formed. Multiple small nodules are seen at irregular intervals along affected shafts. The hair is usually brittle, thin and short (Figures 10.7a,b). It occurs in widespread fashion in Netherton's syndrome in which it is combined with ichthyosis linearis circumflexa, a migrating, annular, red, scaly dermatosis, or sometimes with lamellar ichthyosis or congenital ichthyosiform erythroderma. Associated abnormalities include atopy. Trichorrhexis invaginata appears in infancy but improves spontaneously with age.

Tapered fractures: Tapered fractures resembling pencil points are due to inhibition of nucleic acid and protein synthesis in the hair root. Progressive narrowing of the emerging hair shaft may lead to a fracture near the skin surface, resulting in a detached hair with a tapered, proximal end (Figure 4.5b). This is seen in anagen effluvium occurring as the result of a cytostatic drug. Hair growth resumes after withdrawal of the drug resulting in an attached hair with distal tapering. Tapering is also seen in localized areas following radiotherapy and also in alopecia areata. Tapered hairs may also occur in severe protein calorie malnutrition, such as marasmus or kwashiorkor.

Trichoptilosis: Trichoptilosis is longitudinal splitting of the distal end of the hair causing the common split ends or frizzies (Figure 2.14). It is caused by trauma and may occur in excessive weathering or from damage caused by trichotillomania, pruritic dermatoses, or excessive hair styling. It is frequently seen in pili torti, monilethrix, trichothiodystrophy, and trichorrhexis invaginata.

Irregularities of the Hair Shaft

Longitudinal ridging and grooving: Longitudinal ridges and grooves can occur along the hair shaft and are usually covered by intact cuticle. They are commonly present in normal hair but may be seen in various conditions such as congenital hypotrichosis of the Marie-Unna type, and also in pili torti, pili bifurcati, uncombable hair syndrome, trichothiodystrophy, and the loose anagen syndrome. Fine fluting can occur in pili annulati. Vertical grooving of the internodes may be present in monilethrix.

Uncombable hair or pili trianguli et canaliculi: Uncombable hair syndrome is characterized by hair shafts that are usually triangular or kidney shaped in cross section. Longitudinal grooves are present. The hair usually has a silvery-blond color and glitters as the result of reflection and refraction of incident light by the different-shaped hair shafts (Figures 10.8a,b). It is usually noticed at about three years and spontaneous improvement has been seen in some cases in later life.

Loose anagen syndrome: This usually occurs in young children between the ages of three and five and is often seen in fair-haired girls. The hair is easily extractable and this is due to some weakness in the root sheath permitting anagen hairs to be extracted easily and without pain. There may be spontaneous improvement in later life. The loose anagen hair usually lacks a root sheath, has a ruffled cuticle, and may show longitudinal grooving (Figures 10.9a,b,c).

Pili multigemini: In pili multigemini from two to eight hair papillae and matrices with separate internal root sheaths form hairs that emerge from one follicular canal. The hairs are flattened and triangular in cross section and may show longitudinal grooves. They usually emerge as a tuft of individual hairs but readhesion may occur.

(continued)

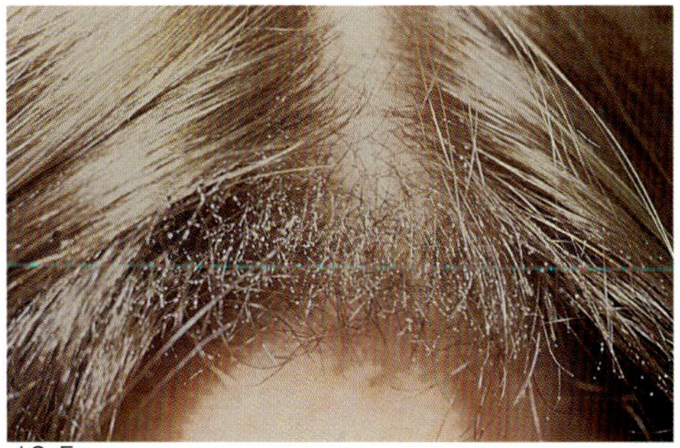
10.5a →

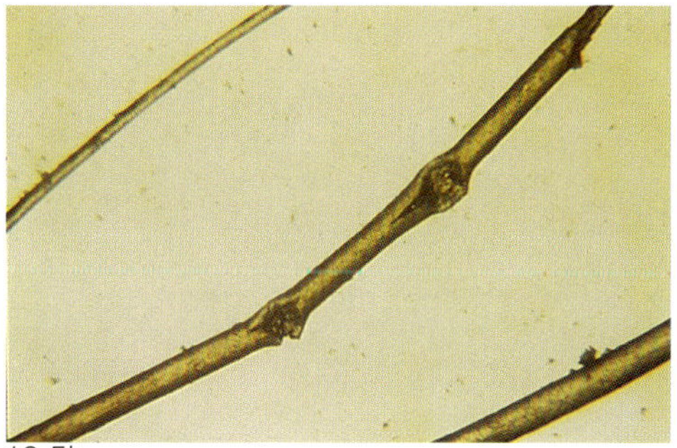
10.5b ■

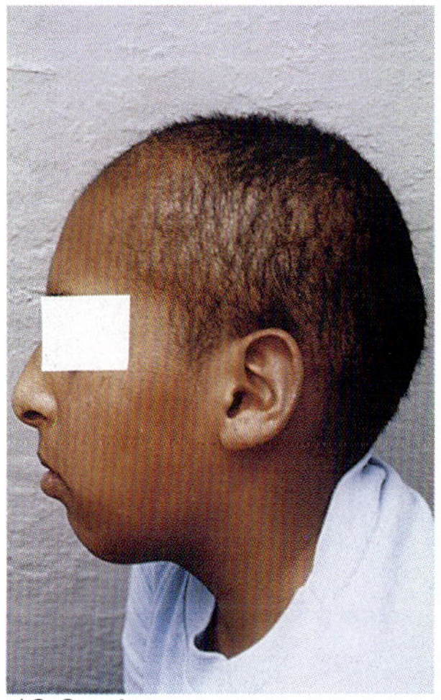
10.6a ↓

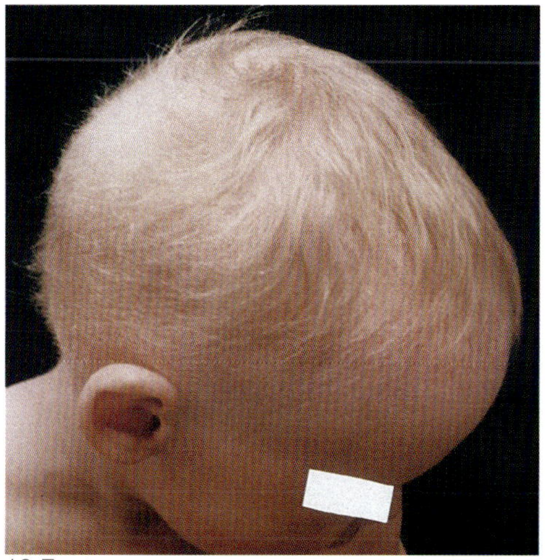
10.7a ↓

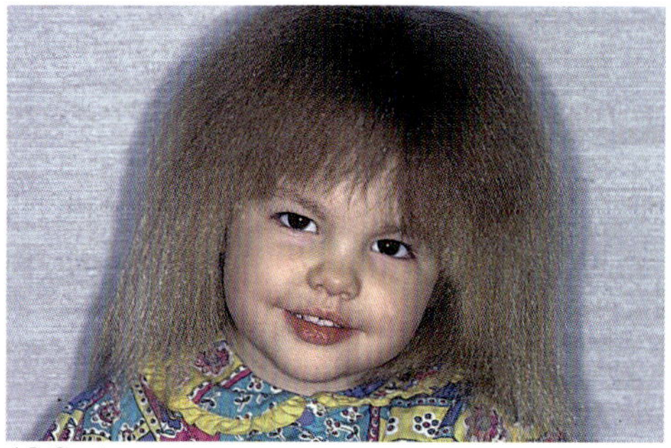
10.8a ↓

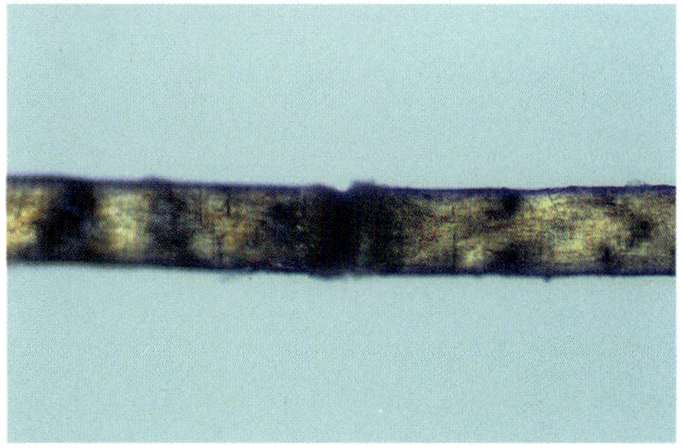
10.6b ■

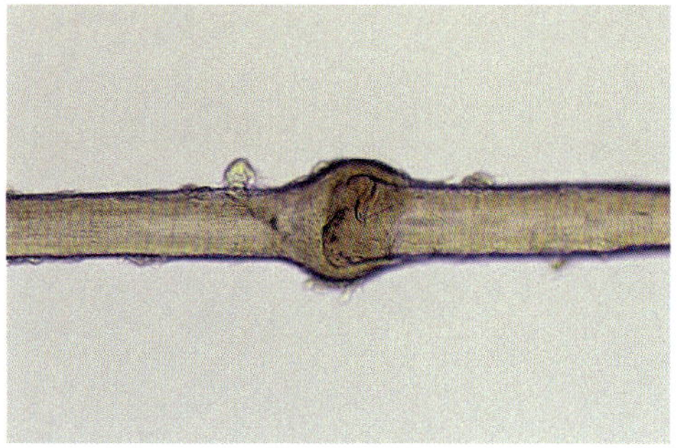
10.7b ■

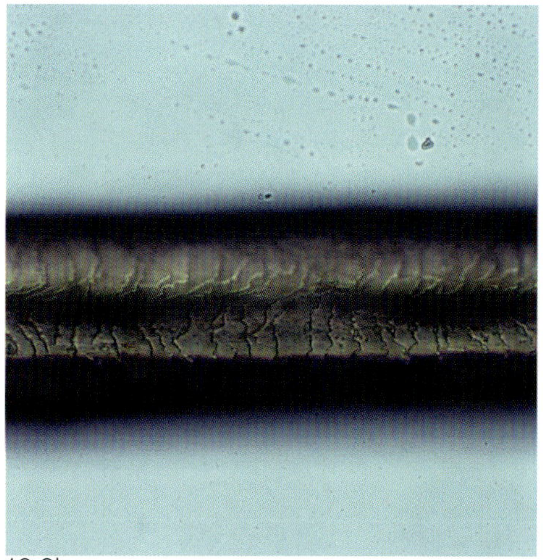
10.8b ■

10.5
Trichorrhexis nodosa:

a. Distal trichorrhexis nodosa from frequent brushing.

b. Microscopic appearances: Typical expanded fractures of trichorrhexis nodosa are seen. LM x 75. *(Reprinted with permission, Whiting, D.A., J. Am. Acad. Dermatol., 1987.)*

10.6
Trichothiodystrophy:

a. A diffuse alopecia from the brittle hair is seen. *(Courtesy of V.H. Price, M.D.)*

b. Microscopic appearances: Polarized light: Clean transverse fracture of trichoschisis is seen with alternating light and dark bands along the shaft. LM x 100.

10.7
Trichorrhexis invaginata:

a. Diffuse alopecia associated with the brittle hairs is present. *(Courtesy of V.H. Price, M.D.)*

b. Microscopic appearances: A ball and socket joint typical of the bamboo hair seen in Netherton's syndrome is present. LM x 100.*(Reprinted with permission, Whiting, D.A., Hair shaft defects, in Disorders of Hair Growth: Diagnosis and Treatment, Olsen, E. A. [Ed]. McGraw-Hill, 1994).*

10.8
Uncombable hair:

a. Typical uncombable hair with a silvery sheen surrounds this patient's scalp.

b. Microscopic appearances: A longitudinal groove is present with normal cuticular pattern. LM x 400.

Pili annulati: Pili annulati or ringed hair shows characteristic alternating bright and dark bands on the hair shaft on light microscopy. It may be present at birth or appear during infancy and is usually familial.

Monilethrix: In monilethrix the hair show an irregular, beaded appearance due to elliptical expansions of the hair shaft at approximately 1-mm intervals. There may be longitudinal grooving at the internodes and loss of cuticle cells over the nodes from weathering. There is no medullary cavity in the internodes. The abnormally brittle hairs break at the internodes. It appears in early childhood mostly on the occiput and nape but can affect the entire scalp and even the facial and general body hair. The beaded hairs emerge from keratotic follicular papules and rarely grow longer than 1 to 2 cm (Figures 10.10a,b). Some improvement may occur in later life. Monilethrix is of dominant inheritance and can be associated with physical retardation, juvenile cataracts, and other abnormalities of nails and teeth.

Bubble hairs: Bubble hairs are characterized by rows of bubbles within the hair shaft. No obvious abnormality of the hair cuticle is present (Figures 10.11a,b). The bubbles are caused by overheating of the hair shaft by a hair dryer which is set too high. The condition clears spontaneously.

Hair Shaft Coiling and Twisting

Pili torti: In pili torti the hair shaft is flattened and twisted from 90 to 360 degrees on its own axis. Four or five twists are found at irregular intervals along the hair shaft. The cuticle cells are intact. The hairs are brittle and usually fracture within the twists. Classical pili torti is usually found in association with thin, blond hairs and occurs in early childhood commencing on the occipital and temporal regions and sometimes involving eyebrows and eyelashes (Figures 10.12a,b). It often improves after puberty but may persist. It can be associated with dental abnormalities, nail dystrophy, corneal opacities, sensorineural deafness, keratosis pilaris, and ichthyosis. Females are predominantly affected. A postpubertal type of pili torti associated with mental retardation affects both sexes. Pili torti has been reported with various other abnormalities. Corkscrew hair is a rare type of pili torti, with a double twist in some hairs, alopecia, and an associated ectodermal dysplasia (Figures 10.13a,b).

Woolly hair: Woolly hairs are similar to the common Negroid hair form and are tightly coiled with an average curl diameter of 0.5 cm. Woolly hair may be hereditary, or familial and sporadic, or may occur as a woolly hair nevus. The hair shafts show a variable number of 180-degree axial twists. The hairs are usually ovoid in cross section and usually show no other abnormality. However, in woolly hair nevus the hairs may show irregularities of the

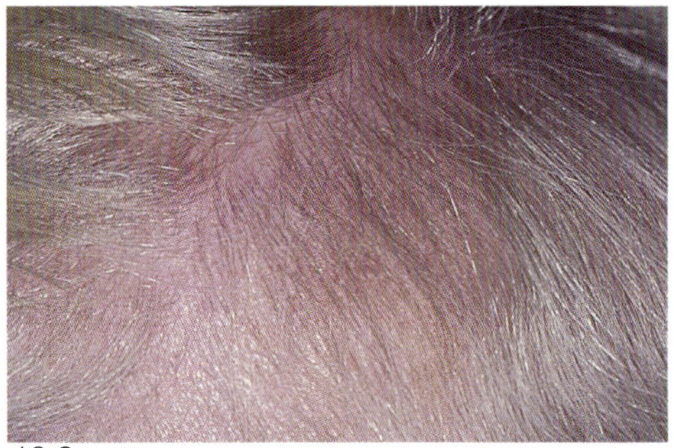
10.9a →

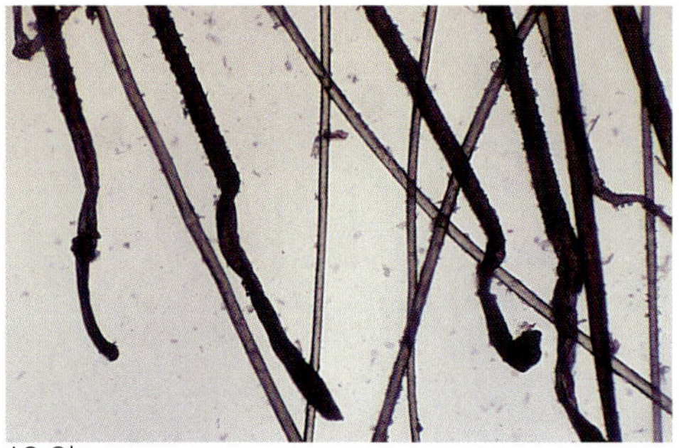
10.9b →

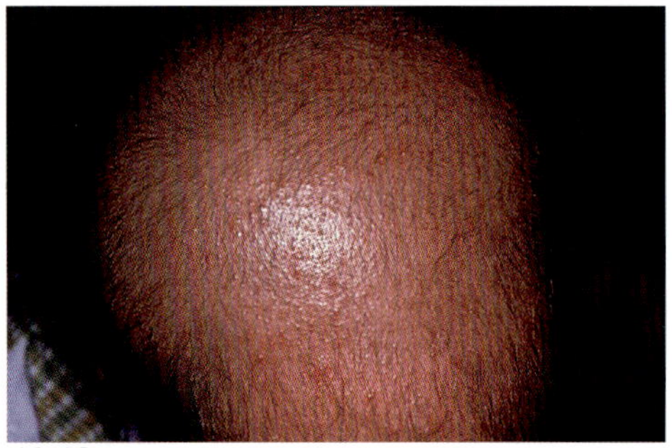
10.10a →

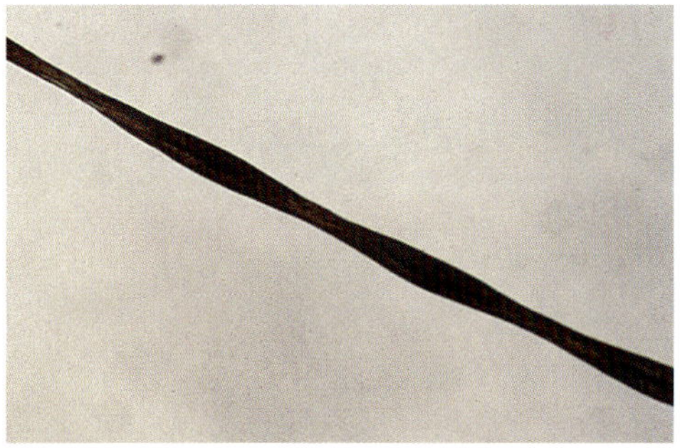
10.10b ■

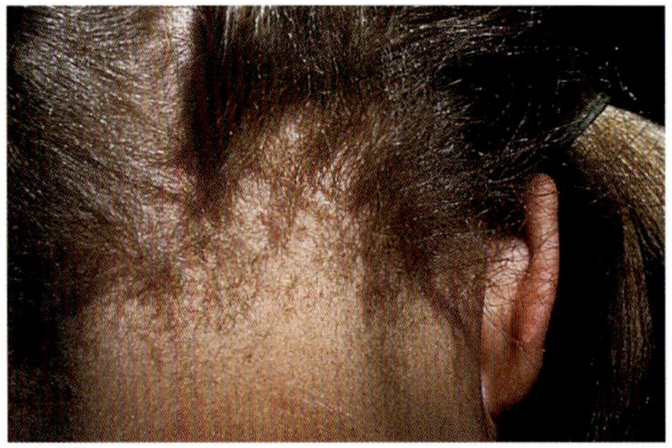
10.12a →

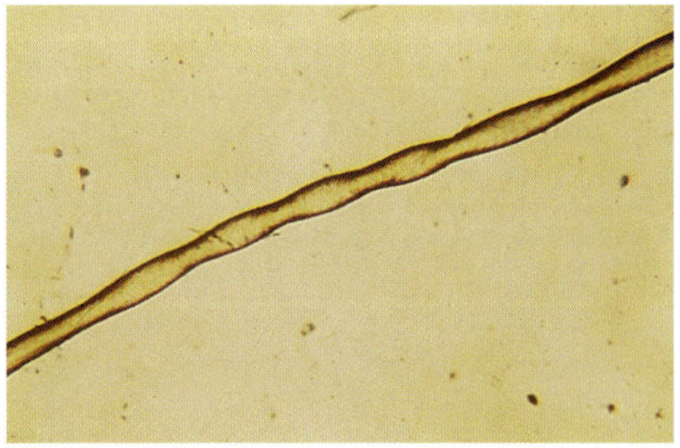
10.12b ■

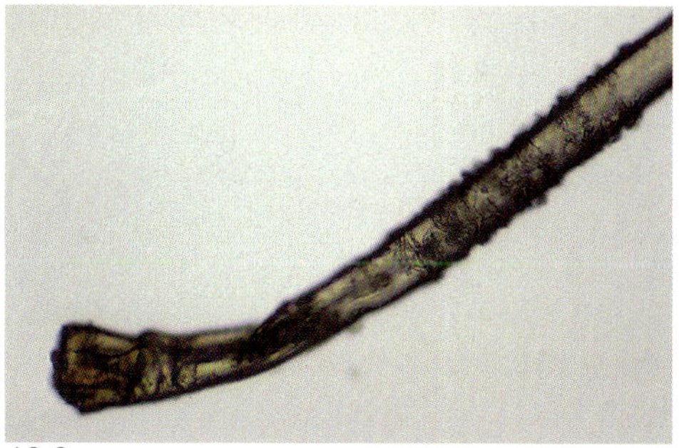
10.9c ■

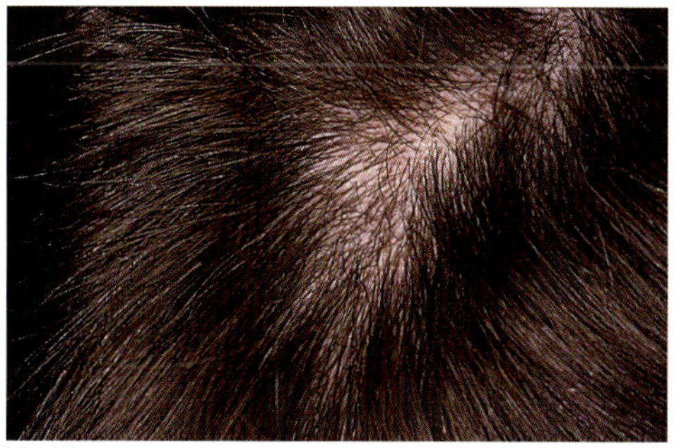
10.11a →

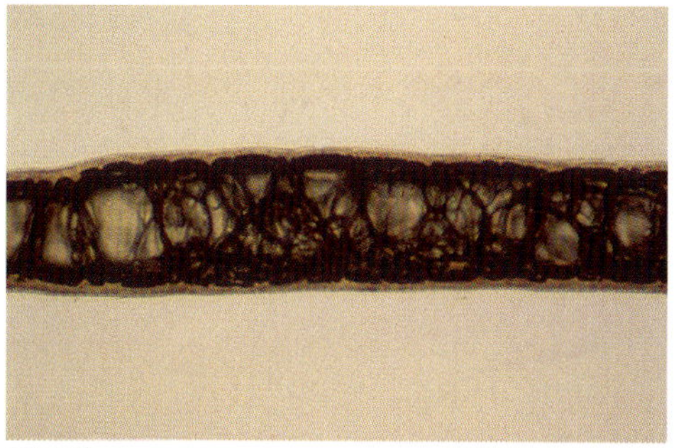
10.11b ■

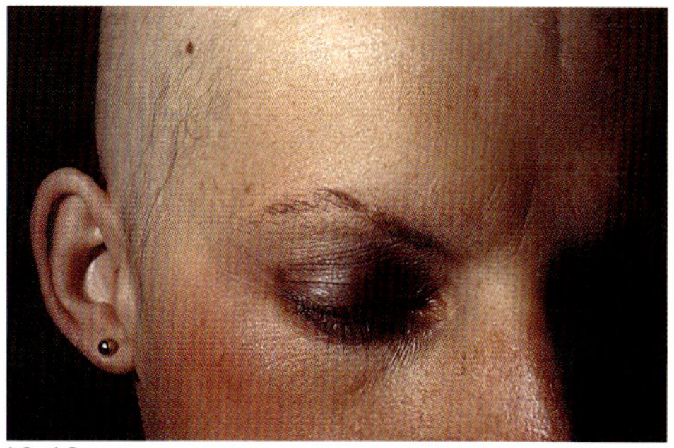
10.13a →

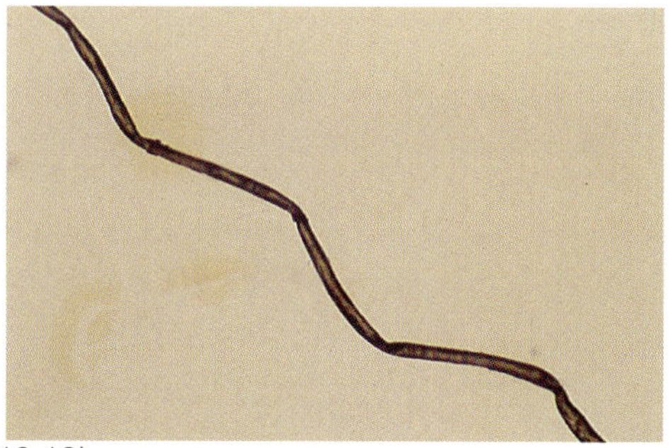
10.13b ■

10.9
Loose anagen syndrome:

a. Patchy hair loss is present in a blond child.

b. Microscopic appearances: A clump of easily extracted anagen hairs is shown here. LM x 40.

c. Microscopic appearances: Anagen hair root is seen here lacking a root sheath and showing a ruffled cuticle and longitudinal groove. LM x 100. *(Reprinted with permission, Whiting, D.A., Hair shaft defects, in Disorders of Hair Growth: Diagnosis and Treatment, Olsen, E. A. [Ed]. McGraw-Hill, 1994).*

10.10
Monilethrix:

a. Severe alopecia from monilethrix associated with keratosis pilaris-like appearance. *(Reprinted with permission, Whiting, D.A., Hair shaft defects, in Disorders of Hair Growth: Diagnosis and Treatment, Olsen, E. A. [Ed]. McGraw-Hill, 1994).*

b. Microscopic appearances: Regular beading of the hair shaft is seen. LM x 40.

10.11
Bubble hair:

a. A small patch of alopecia is shown containing some distorted hairs.

b. Microscopic appearances: The hair shaft is distended by rows of bubbles. LM x 100. *(Reprinted with permission, Whiting, D.A., Hair shaft defects, in Disorders of Hair Growth: Diagnosis and Treatment, Olsen, E. A. [Ed]. McGraw-Hill, 1994).*

10.12
Pili torti:

a. Twisted hairs are present over the occiput in this blond child aged 5 years.*(Reprinted with permission, Whiting, D.A., Hair shaft defects, in Disorders of Hair Growth: Diagnosis and Treatment, Olsen, E. A. [Ed]. McGraw-Hill, 1994).*

b. Microscopic appearances: Irregular 180 degree twists are present in the hair shaft. LM x 40.*(Reprinted with permission, Whiting, D.A., Hair shaft defects, in Disorders of Hair Growth: Diagnosis and Treatment, Olsen, E. A. [Ed]. McGraw-Hill, 1994).*

10.13
Corkscrew hair:

a. Severe alopecia with some scattered hairs is present (accompanied by enamel hypoplasia and webbed toes).

b. Microscopic appearances: The zigzag appearance of this hair is due to a double twist superimposed on an underlying pili torti. LM x 40. *(Reprinted with permission, Whiting, D.A., Jenkins, T., Whitcomb, M.J., Hair, Trace Elements, and Human Illness, Praeger, 1980.)*

hair shaft (Figures 10.14a,b). 50% of cases of woolly hair nevus are associated with a linear nevus on the neck or arms and ocular abnormalities may be present.

Acquired progressive kinking: Acquired progressive kinking of the hair appears in the late teens or early twenties with gradual symmetric curling and darkening of the hair in the frontal, temporal and auricular areas (Figures 10.15a,b,c). Some cases may progress to androgenetic alopecia but others may improve spontaneously.

Trichonodosis: Trichonodosis or knotting of the hair shaft can occur as single or double knots. Secondary changes in the vicinity include cuticular loss with possible fractures of the shaft. It is caused by trauma and traction from cosmetic procedures and from friction from pillows and occurs mostly in short curly hair.

Extraneous Matter on Hair Shaft

Fungi: Dermatophytes (Figures 9.1a,b, 9.3a,b) and black and white piedra can affect and damage hair shafts (see Chapter 9).

Bacteria: Trichomycosis axillaris is caused by *Corynebacterium tenuis* which forms adherent yellow or orange nodules around affected hairs (see Chapter 9).

Pediculosis capitis: In pediculosis capitis the nits are often easier to find than are the adult lice. On the scalp both nits and lice are most numerous on the occiput and behind the ears. The typical oval nit or oval egg case is attached securely to the hair and lies to one side of it. The free distal end of the nit points towards the hair tip (Figures 9.14a,b) (see Chapter 9).

Peripilar casts: Peripilar casts or pseudonits are commonly found in normal hair, especially in female children. They are whitish or yellowish in color and are easily moved along the hair shaft which pierces the cast centrally. True peripilar keratin casts are usually composed of external root sheath, rarely of internal root sheath, and sometimes of both (Figure 10.16).

Deposits: Lacquer, paint (Figure 10.17), glue and other chemicals (Figure 10.18) may be deposited on the hair shafts and may cause diagnostic difficulty. Deposits are localized to the areas of contact.

Histopathology

Histopathology is usually not necessary in the diagnosis of hair shaft abnormalities. It can however be useful in diagnosing underlying alopecia areata, trichotillomania, and other dermatoses. It can also be useful in recognizing triangular or kidney shaped transverse sections of hair shafts in uncombable hair and may also be useful in diagnosing pili multigemini or bifurcarti.

Investigation and Diagnosis

Hair samples for light microscopy are easily mounted in parallel on glass slides previously coated with double-stick clear tape or with two fresh bands of an appropriate mounting medium. Hair shaft abnormalities should be found consistently in samples from different areas of the scalp in order to be considered significant. Hair specimens are obtained with a pull test by gentle extraction with the fingers or by cutting the hairs off next to the scalp with sharp scissors. Forcible extraction using a needle holder is not recommended routinely due to the variety of artifactual changes produced in the hair root and shaft. Hair shaft abnormalities can usually be diagnosed in the office by light microscopy. Scanning electron microscopy is useful in confirming the diagnosis of uncombable hair. Careful examination for other abnormalities of skin, hair, nails and teeth is necessary.

Differential Diagnosis

Final diagnosis depends on correlation of the hair shaft abnormality with other clinical signs. A careful history is also necessary here. Remember that certain hair shaft abnormalities are produced by trauma and can occur in many different conditions.

Treatment

Treatment depends upon the cause. In general it is important to make hair styling as gentle as possible. ■

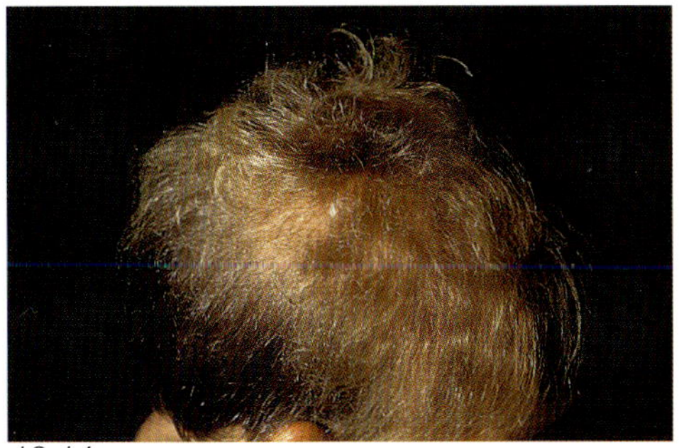
10.14a →

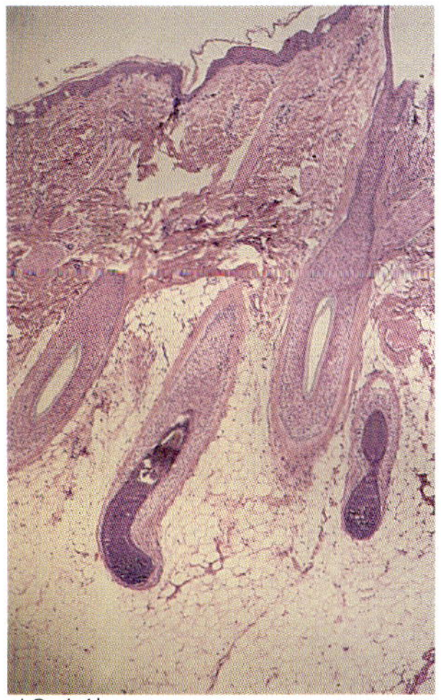
10.14b ■

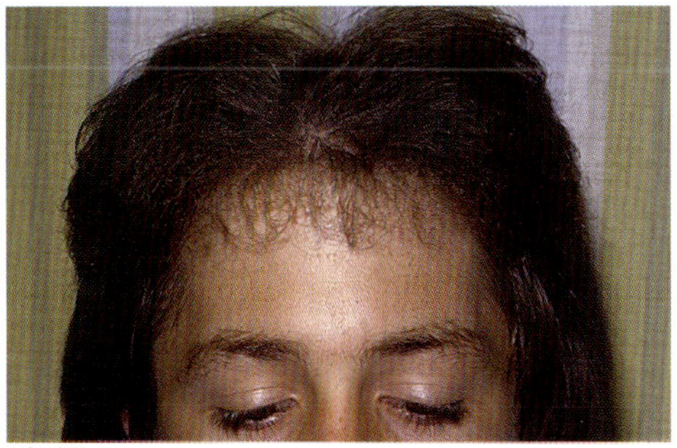
10.15a →

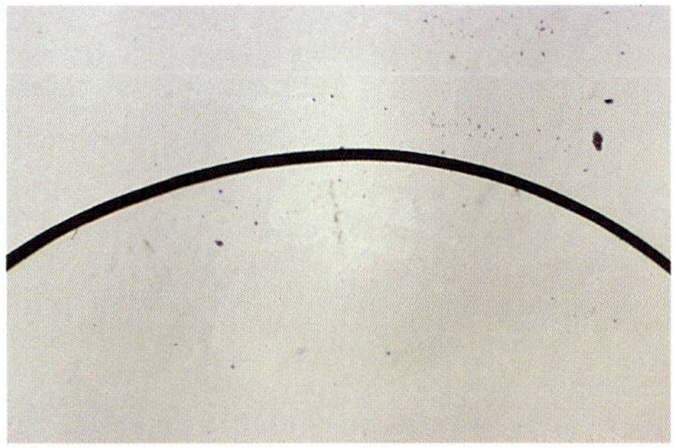
10.15b →

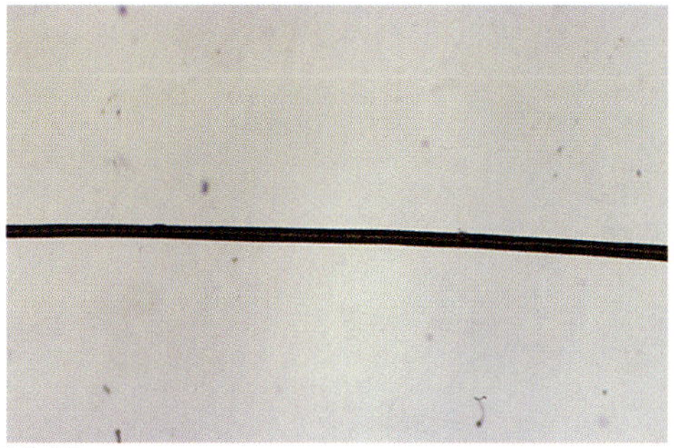
10.15c ■

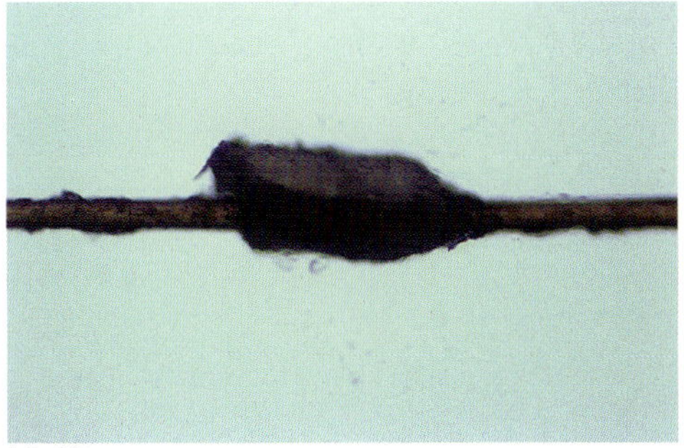
10.16

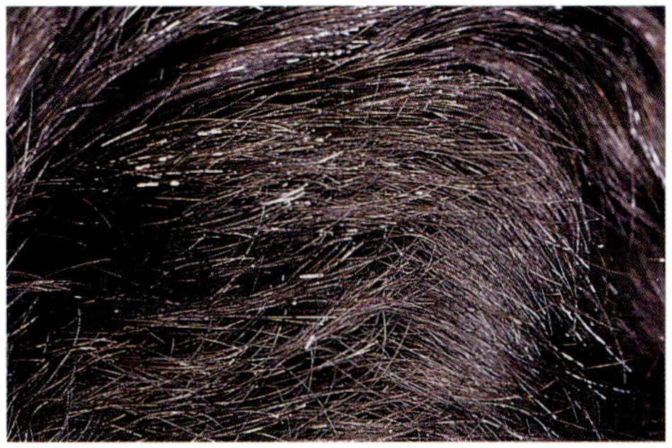
10.17

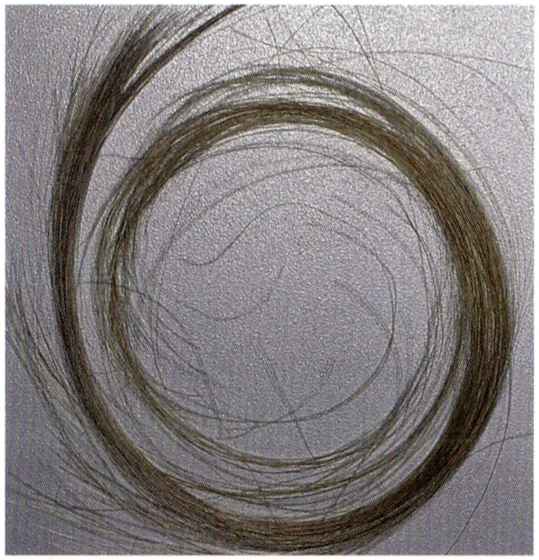
10.18

10.14
Woolly hair nevus:

a. Fair woolly hair represents the nevus and the dark hair is the normal. *(Reprinted with permission, Whiting, D.A., J. Am. Acad. Dermatol., 1987.)*

b. Scalp biopsy: Histopathology of woolly hair nevus: Vertical section: A right angle curve is present in the lower hair follicle, presumably accounting for the hair shaft irregularity. LM x 40.

10.15
Acquired progressive kinking:

a. Kinky hair has recently developed on the forehead and temples of this teenager.*(Reprinted with permission, Whiting, D.A., Hair shaft defects, in Disorders of Hair Growth: Diagnosis and Treatment, Olsen, E. A. [Ed]. McGraw-Hill, 1994).*

b. A kinked hair. LM x 40.

c. A straight normal hair from the same patient. LM x 40.

10.16
Peripilar cast: A cast composed of external root sheath is seen here. LM x 100.

10.17
Extraneous matter on the hair shaft: White paint is seen coating some of the hairs here.

10.18
Green hair: The greenish discoloration was caused by corrosion of copper pipes supplying a swimming pool.

Recommended Reading

Aoyagi, T., Porter, P.S.: "Genetic disorders of hair growth: pathogenesis of human hair defects." In: Kobori, T., Montagna, W., Toda, K. (Eds.) *Biology and disease of the hair.* Baltimore: University Park Press. 1976:473–487.

Beare, J.M.: "Congenital pilar defect showing features of pili torti." *Br J Dermatol* 1952;64:366–372.

Bentley-Phillips, B., Bayles, M.A.H.: "Pseudo monilethrix." *Br J Dermatol* 1975;92:113–115.

Brown, U.M., Crounse, R.G., Abele, D.C.: "An unusual new hair shaft abnormality: 'Bubble hair.'" *J Am Acad Dermatol* 1986;15:1113–1117.

Chernosky, M.E., Owens, D.W.: "Trichorrhexis nodosa. Clinical and investigative studies." *Arch Dermatol* 1966;94:577–585.

Coupe, R.L., Johnston, M.M.: "Acquired progressive kinking of the hair. Structural changes and growth dynamics of affected hairs." *Arch Dermatol* 1969;100:191–195.

Crandall, B.G., Samec, L., Sparkes, R.S., et al.: "A familial syndrome of deafness, alopecia, and hypogonadisim." *J Pediatr* 1973;82:461–465.

Dawber, R.P.R.: "Knotting of scalp hair." *Br J Dermatol* 1974;91:169–173.

de Berker, D., Dawber, R.P.R.: "Monilethrix: clinical and microscopic findings in 21 cases." *Br J Dermatol* 1991;125: Suppl.38, 24.

Detwiler, S.P., Carson, J.L., Woosley, J.T., et al.: "Bubble hair: Case caused by an overheating hair dryer and reproducibility in normal hair with heat." *J Am Acad Dermatol* 1994;30:54–60.

Eckert, J., Church, R.E., Ebling, F.J.: "The pathogensis of alopecia areata." *Br J Dermatol* 1968;80:203–210.

Greene, S.L., Muller, S.A.: "Netherton's syndrome." *J Am Acad Dermatol* 1985;13:329–337.

Hutchinson, P.E., Cairns, R.J., Wells, R.S.: "Woolly hair. Clinical and genetic aspects." *Trans St. John's Hosp Dermatol Soc* 1974;60:160–177.

Itin, P.H., Pittlekow, M.R.: "Trichothiodystrophy: review of sulfur-deficient brittle hair syndromes and association with ectodermal dysplasias." *J Am Acad Dermatol* 1990;22:705–717.

Ito, M., Ito, K., Hashimoto, K.: "Pathogenesis in trichorrhexis invaginata (bamboo hair)." *J Invest Dermatol* 1984;83:1–6.

Kalter, D.C., Tschen, J.A., Cernoch, P.L., et al.: "Genital white piedra: epidemiology, microbiology and therapy." *J Am Acad Dermatol* 1986;14:982–993.

Keifert, J.A.: "Hair casts. Review and suggestion regarding nomenclature." *Arch Dermatol* 1986;122:927–930.

Kligman, A.M.: "Tinea capitis due *M. audouini* and *M. canis*." *Arch Dermatol* 1955;71:313–357.

Kurwa, A.R., Abdel-Aziz, A.M.: "Pili torti – congenital and acquired." *Acta Derm Venereol (Stockh)* 1973;53:385–392.

McBride, M.E., Freeman, R.G., Knox, J.M.: "The bacteriology of trichomycosis axillaris." *Br J Dermatol* 1968;80:509–513.

Mehregan, A.H., Thompson, W.S.: "Pili multigemini. Report of a case in association with cleidocranial dyostosis." *Br J Dermatol* 1979;100:315–322.

Menkes, J.H.: "Kinky hair disease." *Pediatrics* 1972;50:181–183.

Mortimer, P.S.: "Unruly hair." *Br J Dermatol* 1985;113:467–473.

Muller, S.: "Alopecia: syndromes of genetic significance." *J Invest Dermatol* 1973;60:475–492.

Peachey, R.D.G., Wells, R.S.: "Hereditary hypotrichosis (Marie Unna type)." *Trans St. John's Hosp Dermatol Soc* 1971;57:157–166.

Porter, P.S., Lobitz, W.C.: "Human hair: a genetic marker." *Br J Dermatol* 1970;83:225–241.

Price, V.H.: "Structural anomalies of the hair shaft." In: Orfanos, C.E., Happle, R., eds. *Hair and hair diseases.* Berlin: Springer-Verlag, 1990:363–422.

Price, V.H., Gummer, C.L.: "Loose anagen syndrome." *J Am Acad Dermatol* 1989;20:249–256.

Price, V.H., Odom, R.B., Ward, W.H., et al.: "Trichothiodystrophy. Sulfur-deficient brittle hair as a marker for a neuroectodermal symptom complex." *Arch Dermatol* 1980;116:1375–1384.

Price, V.H., Thomas, R.S., Jones, F.G.: "Pili annulati. Optical and electron microscopic studies." *Arch Dermatol* 1968;98:640–647.

Price, V.H., Thomas, R.S., Jones, F.G.: "Pseudopili annulati: an unusual variant of normal hair." *Arch Dermatol* 1970;102:354–358.

Ronchese, F.: "Twisted hairs (pili torti)." *Arch Dermatol Syphilol* 1932;26:98–109.

Rook, A.: "Review: the clinical importance of "weathering" in human hair." *Br J Dermatol* 1976;95:111–112.

Rook, A., Dawber, R.: *Diseases of the Hair and Scalp.* (2nd ed.) Oxford: Blackwell Scientific Publications. 1991:200–255.

Sims, R.T.: "'Beau's lines' in hair. Reduction of hair shaft diameter associated with illness." *Br J Dermatol* 1967;79:43–49.

Stroud, J.D., Mehregan, A.H.: "'Spun glass' hair: a clinicopathologic study of an unusual hair defect." In: Brown, A.C., (Ed.) *The first human hair symposium.* New York: Medcom 1973;103–107.

Weary, P., Hendricks, A.A., Warner, F., et al.: "Pili bifurcati. A new anomaly of hair growth." *Arch Dermatol* 1973;108:403–407.

Whiting, D.A., Jenkins, T., Whitcomb, M.J: "Corkscrew hair - a unique type of congenital alopecia in pili torti." In Brown, A.C., Crounse, R.G., (Eds.) *Hair, trace elements, and human illness.* New York: Praeger, 1980:228–239.

Whiting, D.A.: "Structural abnormalities of the hair shaft." *J Am Acad Dermatol* 1987;16:1–25.

Whiting, D.A.: "Hair shaft defects." In: *Disorders of Hair Growth: Diagnosis and Treatment,* Olsen, E.A. (Ed.). New York: McGraw-Hill 1994, 91–137.

Wolff, H.H., Vigl, E., Braun-Falco, O.: "Trichorrhexis congenita." *Hautarzt* 1975;26:576–580.

Hereditary and Congenital Alopecia

The classification of hereditary and congenital alopecia will depend upon its extent, whether circumscribed or generalized, its association, or lack thereof, with other abnormalities, and the family history. A complete discussion of such hereditary forms of alopecia is far beyond the scope of this atlas; however, an attempt will be made to include information on many such conditions.

Circumscribed Alopecia in Infancy

Circumscribed alopecia in the newborn can be due to a number of causes. Physiological occipital alopecia is not uncommon and is nonscarring. The circumscribed patch of alopecia is caused by a postnatal wave of telogen hair loss (Figure 11.1). Obstetrical trauma and associated hematomas or lacerations may be followed by temporary hair loss or by scarring (Figure 11.2). Aplasia cutis congenita, the absence of areas of skin at birth, most commonly affects the scalp. This may present as an ulcerative lesion or as a scar at the time of birth. Involved areas lack dermal appendages and therefore often represent permanent areas of alopecia (Figures 11.3, 6.1). While usually small (1-2 cm in diameter) and solitary, very rarely multiple and extensive lesions can be seen.

The presence of epidermal nevi on the scalp is often associated with partial or complete lack of hair. The sebaceous nevus is most commonly present on the scalp and appears as a slightly raised, velvety plaque which may involute during childhood and become much more prominent at puberty (Figures 6.2a,b). Most sebaceous nevi are relatively small (1-2 cm), however may rarely be extensive. Surgical excision is recommended. Later in life various skin tumors, including basal cell epitheliomata, may develop within the nevus.

Triangular alopecia of the temples is represented by small areas where follicles are miniaturized, sparse or absent and may be found on routine scalp examination (Figure 11.4).

Localized alopecia overlying a meningocele has been described. Alopecia areata and tinea capitis are rare in the newborn but can occur.

During early childhood localized cicatricial alopecia may be seen in incontinentia pigmenti and sutural alopecia in Hallermann-Streiff syndrome (mandibulo-oculo-facial dyscephaly).

(continued)

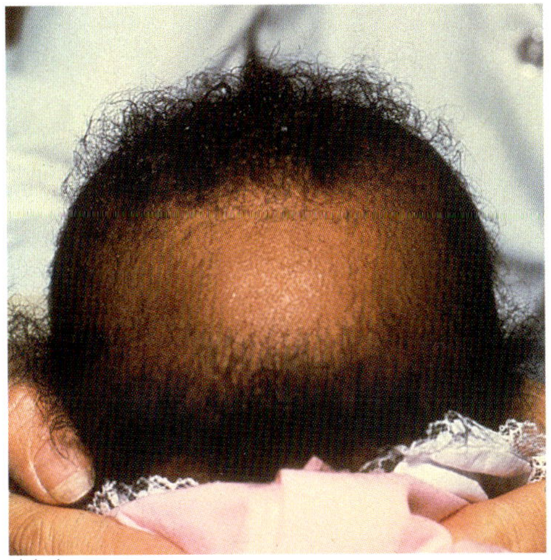
11.1

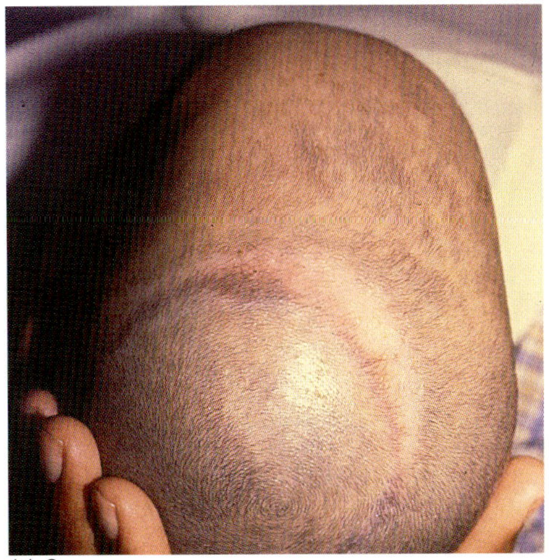
11.2

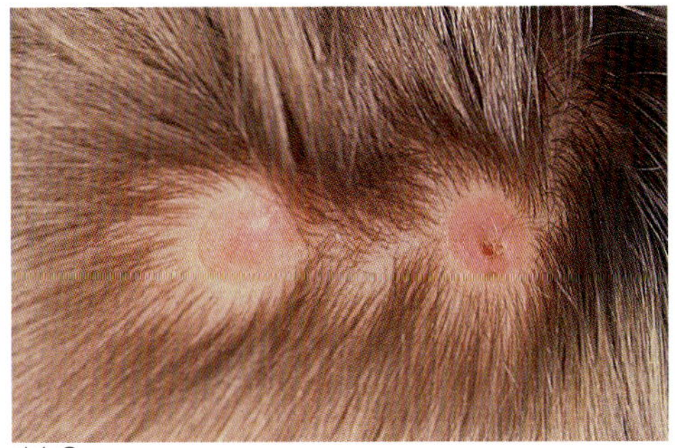
11.3

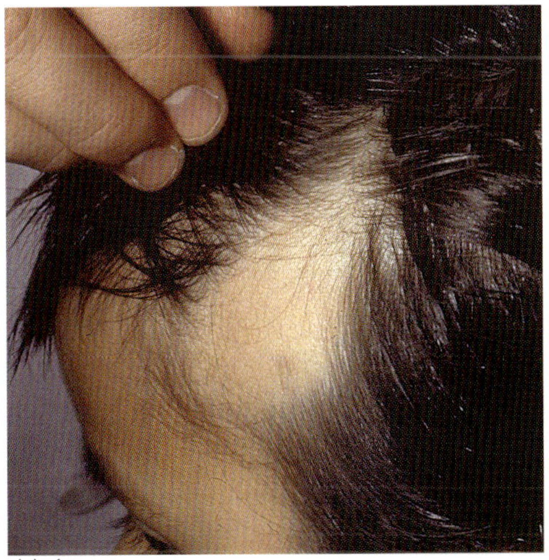
11.4

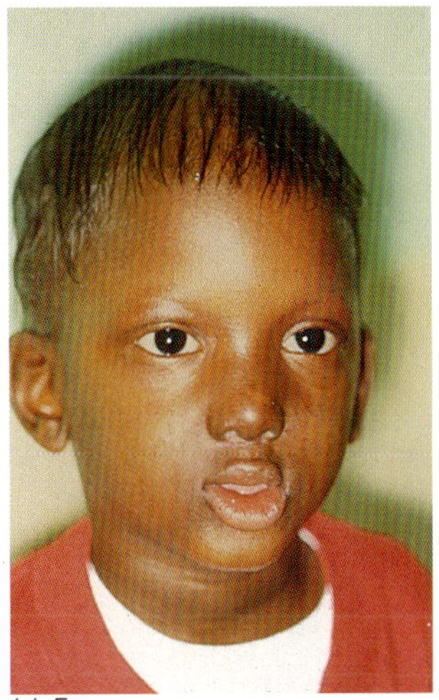
11.5a →

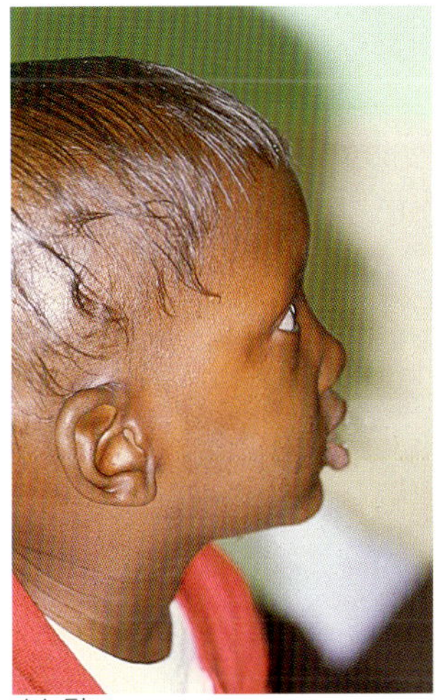
11.5b ■

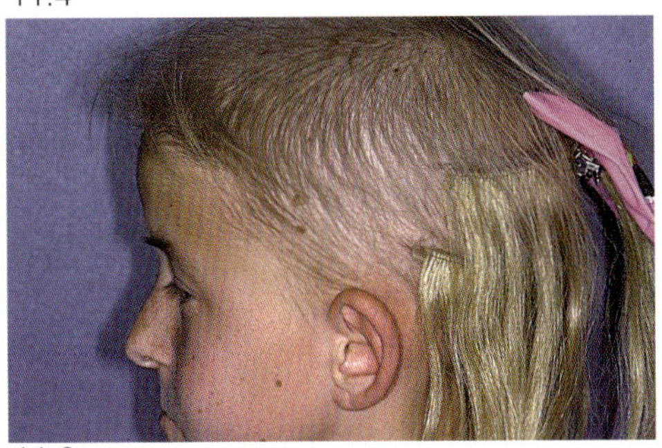
11.6a →

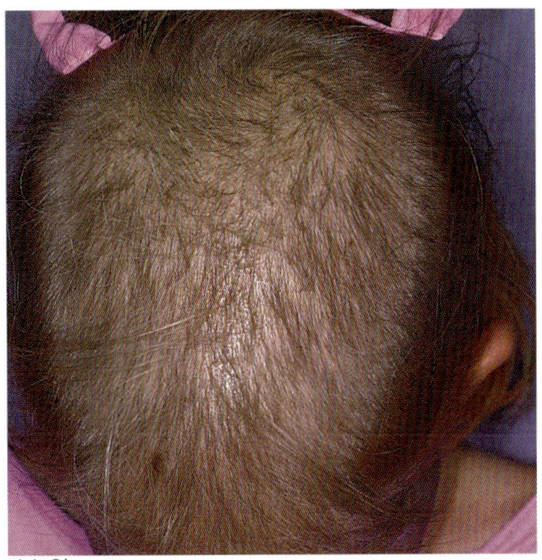
11.6b ■

11.1
Physiological occipital alopecia: Caused by postnatal wave of telogen hair loss.

11.2
Obstetric trauma: "Ventouse" alopecia caused by suction device during delivery. *(Courtesy of H. Francois Jordaan, M. Med.)*

11.3
Aplasia cutis.

11.4
Congenital triangular alopecia, with base of triangle on temporal hairline.

11.5
Anhidrotic ectodermal dysplasia:

a. Frontal view of alopecia with typical facial appearance including saddle nose and pointed chin.

b. Lateral view showing alopecia and prominent forehead.

11.6
Trichorhinophalangeal syndrome:

a. Diffuse alopecia around sides of scalp.

b. Diffuse alopecia over vertex.

Hereditary Diffuse Alopecia and Hypotrichosis

Efforts have been made to classify the hereditary diffuse alopecias. Most have tried to separate such alopecias based on the presence or absence of other associated defects and then in turn the specific type of associated defect. Associated defects generally relate to nails, teeth and sweat gland function. Tables 11.1 through 11.6 provide a summary of many syndromes classified as ectodermal dysplasias which relate to such diffuse alopecia.

Because of the frequent appearance of associated defects with diffuse hereditary alopecia it is essential that evaluation of such alopecia include assessment of teeth, nails and presence or absence of ability to sweat. Any unusual habitus should be noted. Saddle nose, prominent forehead, pointed chin, presence or history of cleft lip or palate, brachydactyly, syndactyly, and other unusual features help define various syndromes.

Certain findings related to major congenital hypotrichosis syndromes without ectodermal defects, or in syndromes associated with premature aging syndromes, or skeletal abnormalities, are detailed in Tables 11.7 through 11.9. Other syndromes in which alopecia is of minor significance are included in Tables 11.10 through 11.12.

Types of inherited diffuse alopecia illustrated here include anhidrotic ectodermal dysplasia (Figures 11.5a,b), trichorhinophalangeal syndrome (Figures 11.6a,b), Langer-Giedion syndrome (Figures 11.7a,b), congenital hypotrichosis (Figures 11.8a,b), hereditary hypotrichosis Marie Unna type (Figures 11.9a,b,c,d), hypomelanosis of Ito (Figure 11.10), and cutis verticis gyrata (Figure 11.11).

The histopathological findings in congenital hypotrichosis include a lack of terminal hairs, but intermediate and "vellus" hairs are present. Increased catagen hairs are seen, with some fibrosis (Figures 11.12a,b). ■

11.7
Langer-Giedion syndrome: Trichorhinophalangeal syndrome with exostosis:

a. Diffuse hair loss is marked in temples.

b. Exostoses add to the irregularities in the fingers.

11.8
Congenital hypotrichosis:

a. Recessive congenital hypotrichosis without associated defects: This patient was bald from birth.

b. Dominant congenital hypotrichosis without associated defects: Mild diffuse thinning of hair in childhood.

11.9
Hereditary hypotrichosis, Marie Unna type:

a,b,c. Diffuse thinning in young adult.

d. Old lady (grandmother) has total alopecia. *(Reprinted with permission, Whiting, D.A., The Diagnosis of Alopecia, Current Concepts, Upjohn, 1990.)*

11.10
Hypomelanosis of Ito: Some diffuse thinning of hair is present.

11.11
Cutis verticis gyrata: Severe diffuse alopecia is present. *(Courtesy of H. Francois Jordaan, M. Med.)*

11.12
Scalp biopsy: Histopathology of congenital hypotrichosis:

a. Vertical section: Terminal hairs are lacking, and only vellus and intermediate hairs are present. LM x 40.

b. Horizontal sections: Several catagen hairs are seen with some surrounding fibrosis. LM x 100.

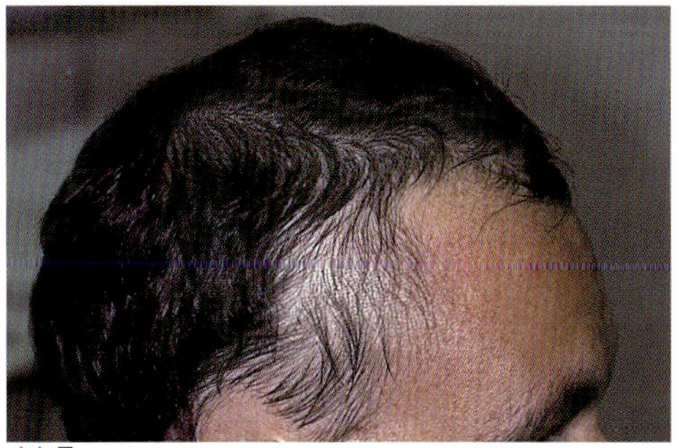
11.7a ➔

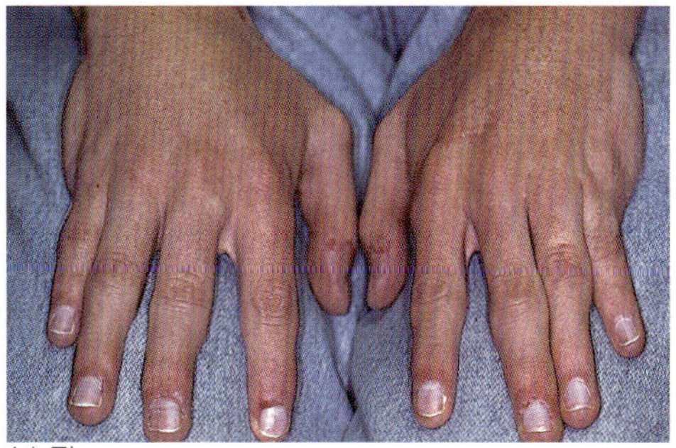
11.7b ■

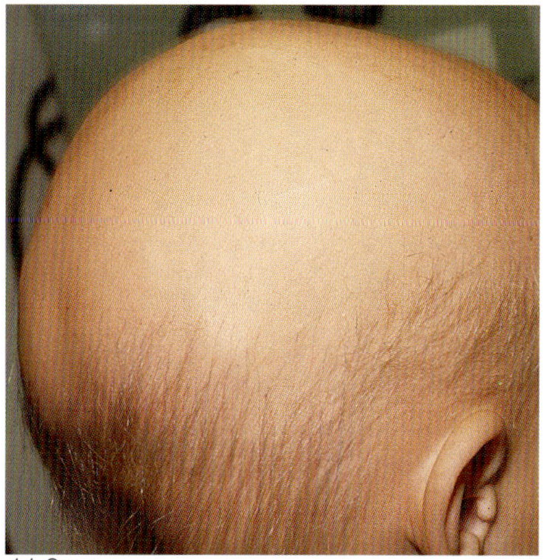
11.8a ➔

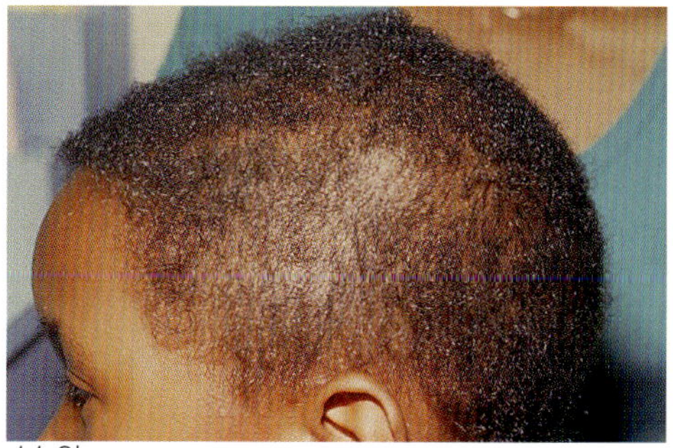
11.8b ■

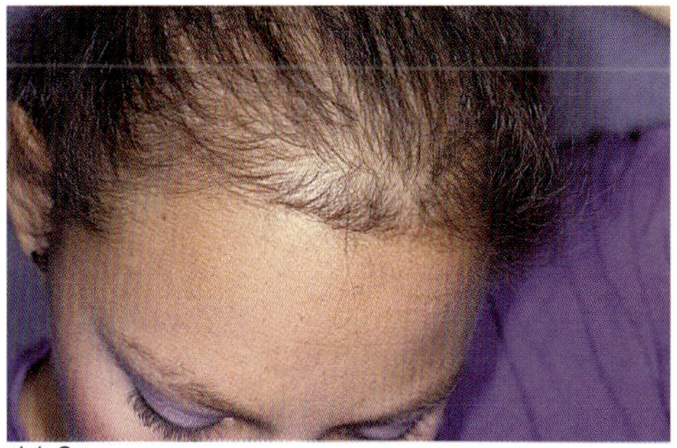
11.9a ➔

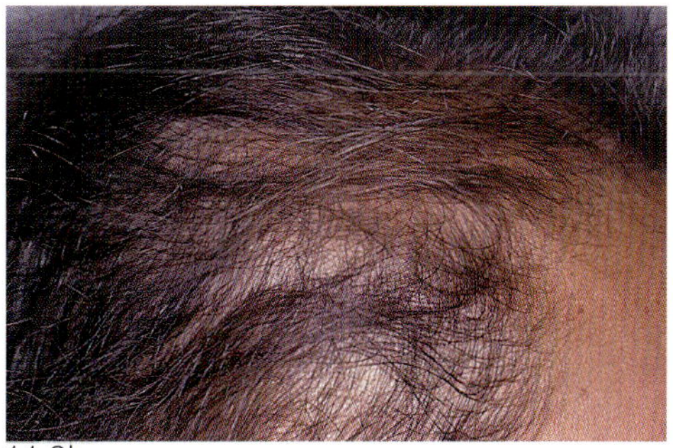
11.9b ➔

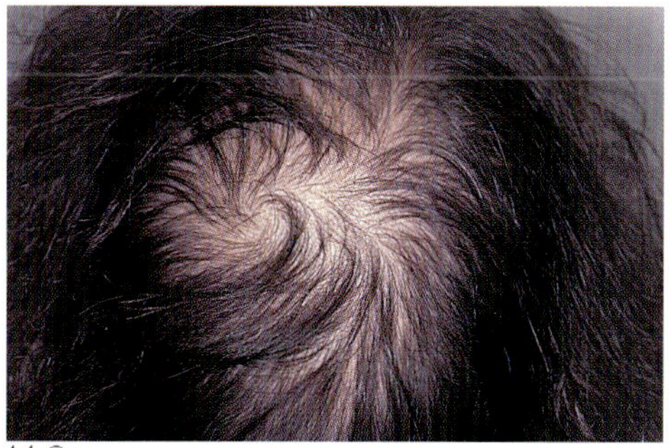
11.9c ➔

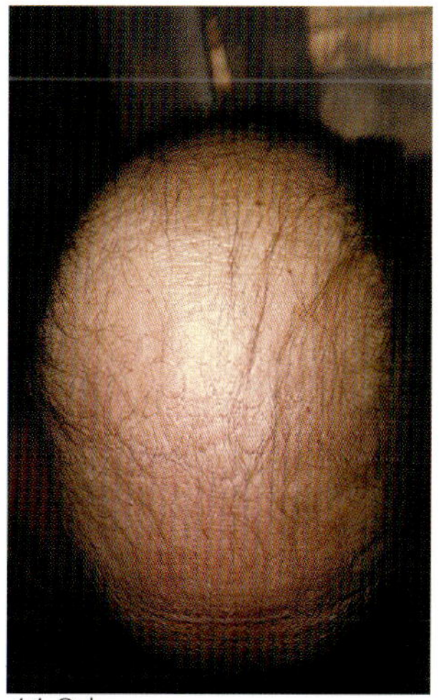
11.9d ■

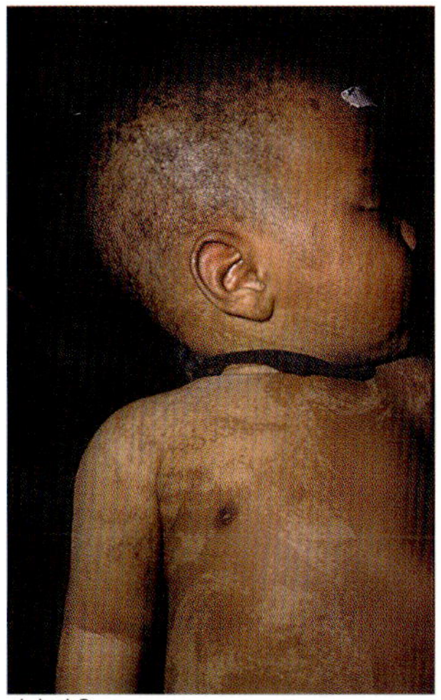
11.10

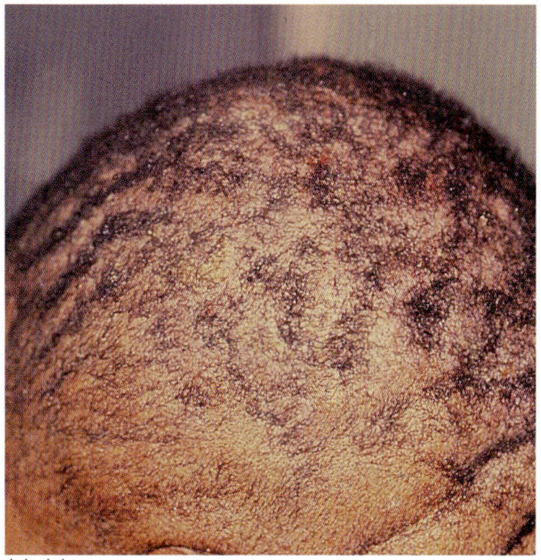
11.11

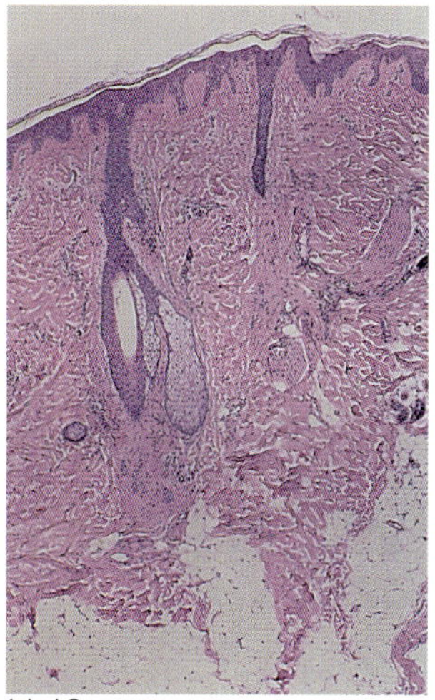
11.12a ➔

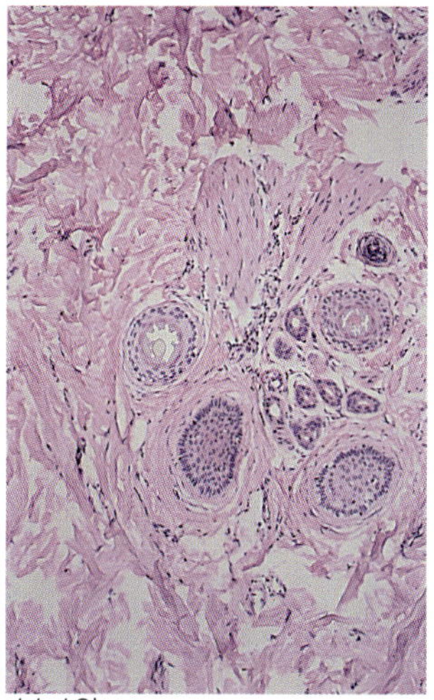
11.12b ■

Table 11.1 Ectodermal Dysplasias – Affecting Hair, Teeth, Nails and Sweat Glands*

Syndrome:	Inheritance	Abnormal Hair	Abnormal Teeth	Abnormal Nails	Abnormal Sweat Glands	Misc.
Anhidrotic ED (Christ–Siemens-Touraine Syndrome)	XR (AR)	Short, fine, sparse and often light in color, eyebrows usually absent	Absent or few, conical canines and incisors discolored and fragile, early caries	Approximately 50% brittle, thin or ridged	Absent or few in number, hyperpyrexia	Prominent forehead, saddle nose, thick lower lip, pointed chin
AEC (Ankyloblepharon, Ectodermal Defects, & Cleft Lip) (Hay-Wells)	AD	Wiry, sparse or absent, longitudinal fluting, focal cuticle defects	Pointed and widely spaced, early caries	Absent or dystrophic	Diminished sweating	Cleft palate/lip, broad nasal bridge, sunken maxilla
Basan	AD	Scalp hair normal early loss during 2nd decade, body hair, eyebrows sparse throughout life	Defective enamel, early caries		Diminished sweating to point of moderate heat intolerance	Dry skin and dry mucous membranes
Ectrodactyly-Ectodermal Dysplasia-Clefting Syndrome (EEC Syndrome)	AD	Sparse, wiry, light colored	Peg–shaped teeth with defective enamel, early caries	Mild dysplasia	Variable-numerous glands on biopsy and sweating may be normal	Lobster claw deformity, cleft lip/palate, lacrimal duct stenosis and corneal scarring
Popliteal Web Syndrome **(Popliteal Pterygium Syndrome)**	AD	Brittle, short, sparse, and light colored	Hypodontia, enamel defects	Toe nail dysplasia	Variable	Cleft palate/lip, lip pits, genital and perineal defects

Table 11.1 continued

Syndrome:	Inheritance	Abnormal Hair	Abnormal Teeth	Abnormal Nails	Abnormal Sweat Glands	Misc.
Rapp-Hodgkin Hypohidrotic Ectodermal Dysplasia	AD	Sparse and light in color associated with pili torti, scarce eyebrows and eyelashes	Conical teeth and hypodentia, early caries	Narrow and dystrophic, hypoplastic	Hypohidrosis severe enough to cause hyperpyrexia	Short, cleft lip/palate and hypospadias high fore-head, narrow nose and small mouth, corneal opacities
Tooth and Nail (Ellis-Dawber Syndrome)	AD	Sparse with some twisting	Peg shaped non–perm. teeth, agenesis of permanent teeth	Hypoplastic	Normal on trunk and limbs, some decrease of palmar sweating sweat duct patency	
Trichodento-Osseous Syndrome (TDO)	AD	Curly at birth, later becomes straighter, curly eyelashes	Small, pitted and widely spaced, early caries		Normal	Frontal bossing, square jaw and long skull
XTE (Xeroderma, Talipes Enamel Defect)	AD	Coarse and sparse, absent eyelashes	Defective enamel	Dystrophic	Small and few in number	Dry skin blisters at times, club foot

AD = autosomal dominant, AR = autosomal recessive, ED = ectodermal dysplasia, XR = sex–linked recessive
*After Rook, A., Dawber, R.: Diseases of the Hair and Scalp (2nd ed). Oxford: Blackwell Scientific Publications, 1991:167–199.

Table 11.2 Ectodermal Dysplasias – Affecting Hair, Teeth, and Nails*

Syndrome	Inheritance	Abnormal Hair	Abnormal Teeth	Abnormal Nails	Abnormal Sweat Glands	Miscellaneous
Clouston's Hidrotic ED	AD	Very sparse, fine, pale and brittle (may be totally absent), eyebrows and lashes sparse or absent	Usually normal	Consistently dystrophic, ridged, thickened and discolored, claw-like	Normal sweating	Palmo-plan tar kerato derma (red, scaly and fissured)
Coffin-Siris Syndrome	AD (?AR)	Sparse scalp hair, eyebrows and lashes, hypertri–chosis of limbs, forehead and back	Delayed dentition with small teeth	Abnormal (Predom–inantly fifth finger)	Normal	Abnormalities of phalanges (absence of distal phalanges), broad nose
Ellis-van Creveld (Chondroectodermal Dysplasia)	AR	Sparse hair but may be mild	Oligodontia (attachment of upper lip to gingiva)	Hypoplastic	Normal	Acromegalic dwarfism, 50% congenital heart disease
Schopf Syndrome (Multiple eyelid Hidrocystoma Syndrome)	AR	Marked hypotri–chosis of scalp, sparse and coarse eyebrows/lashes	Hypodontia	Dystrophic	Probably normal	Cysts of eyelid margins (apocrine hidrocystomas) follicular hyperkeratosis
Trichodento-Osseous Syndrome (TDO)	AD	Curly at birth, later becomes straighter curly eyelashes	Small, pitted and widely spaced, early caries		Normal	Frontal bossing, square jaw and long skull

AD = autosomal dominant, AR = autosomal recessive, ED = ectodermal dysplasia
*After Rook, A., Dawber, R.: Diseases of the Hair and Scalp (2nd ed). Oxford: Blackwell Scientific Publications, 1991:167–199.

Table 11.3 Ectodermal Dysplasias – Affecting Hair, Nails and Sweat Glands*

Syndrome	Inheritance	Abnormal Hair	Abnormal Nails	Abnormal Sweat Glands	Miscellaneous
Friere–Maia	AR	Sparse	Dystrophic	Variable	Hyperkeratosis of palms, soles, elbows and knees, deafness

AR = autosomal recessive
*After Rook, A., Dawber, R.: Diseases of the Hair and Scalp (2nd ed). Oxford: Blackwell Scientific Publications, 1991:167–199.

Table 11.4 Ectodermal Dysplasias – Affecting Hair and Nails*

Syndrome	Inheritance	Abnormal Hair	Abnormal Nails	Miscellaneous
Chands (Curly Hair, Ankyloblepharon Nail Dysplasia Syndrome)	AD	Curly hair	Dysplastic	Ankyloblepharon
Onychotrichodysplasia with Neutropenia (Cantu Syndrome)	AR	Sparse	Dystrophic	Mild mental retardation and chronic neutropenia

AD – autosomal dominant, AR – autosomal recessive
*After Rook, A., Dawber, R.: Diseases of the Hair and Scalp (2nd ed). Oxford: Blackwell Scientific Publications, 1991:167–199.

Table 11.5 Ectodermal Dysplasias – Affecting Hair and Teeth*

Syndrome	Inheritance	Abnormal Hair	Abnormal Teeth	Miscellaneous
Oro-facial-digital Syndrome I (Papillon–Leage and Psaume)	XD (lethal in males)	Fine, sparse, dry and dull, patchy or streaks of loss	Lower lateral incisors fail to develop	Cleft palate/lip, lobed tongue, skeletal defects, milia at birth
Sensenbrenner	AR	Short and very fine	Small, grey and widely spaced	Small, dolichocephalic, unusual facies, eversion of lower lip
Trichodental	AD	Fine, dry, luster–less, slow growing, medially thick, laterally thin eyebrows	Hypodontia	

AD = autosomal dominant, AR = autosomal recessive, XD = sex–linked derived
*After Rook, A., Dawber, R.: Diseases of the Hair and Scalp (2nd ed). Oxford: Blackwell Scientific Publications, 1991:167–199.

Table 11.6 Ectodermal Dysplasias – Affecting hair*

Syndrome	Inheritance	Abnormal Hair	Miscellaneous
Dubowitz	AR	Sparse and fine	Distinct facies, mental retardation, eczema
Moynahan (Alopecia–Epilepsy-Oligophrenia syndrome)		Absence of hair at birth, very sparse hair later	Epilepsy, severe mental retardation
Tricho-rhino-phalangeal Type I	AD	Fine, brittle, sparse	Distinct facies with pear–shaped nose, fusinform proximal IP joints
Tricho-rhino-phalangeal Type II (Langer-Giedion)	Sporadic	Sparse	Bulbous nose, thin upper lip, large protruding ears, exostoses, loose skin

AD = autosomal dominant, AR = autosomal recessive

*After Rook, A., Dawber, R.: Diseases of the Hair and Scalp (2nd ed). Oxford: Blackwell Scientific Publications, 1991:167–199.

Table 11.7 Major Congenital Hypotrichosis in Hereditary Syndromes*

	Inheritance	Abnormal Hair	Miscellaneous
Atrichia with Papular Lesions	AR	Bald from birth or shortly thereafter with subsequent development of follicular cysts (pin-head sized) by age 5-7 yrs	Dental defects and retarded ossification have been reported in some cases
Hallermann-Streiff Syndrome (Mandibulo-Oculo-Facial Dyscephaly)	Sporadic (may be AD)	Normal at birth but soon becomes sparse and brittle with baldness of scalp margins and following cranial sutures	Beaked nose, hypoplastic mandible (bird-like) ocular defects, dental defects
Hereditary Hypotrichosis (Marie Unna)	AD	Usually normal at birth, sparse and twisted later, progressive loss after puberty. Eyebrows/lashes and body hair sparse	Scanty eyebrows and body hair, scarring alopecia. Folliculitis decalvans. Affected individuals otherwise normal

AD = autosomal dominant, AR = autosomal recessive
*After Rook, A., Dawber, R.: Diseases of the Hair and Scalp (2nd ed). Oxford: Blackwell Scientific Publications, 1991:167–199.

Table 11.8 Major Congenital Hypotrichosis in Premature Aging Syndrome*

	Inheritance	Abnormal Hair	Miscellaneous
Bird-Headed Dwarfism (Seckel's Syndrome)	Probably AR	Premature greying and hale patterned loss	Distinctive bird-like facies (beaked nose, micrognathia and low-set ears) dwarfism and microcephaly
Cockayne's Syndrome	AR	Scalp hair normal to fine and sparse, sometimes premature greying	Appear normal at birth, facial erythema in butterfly distribution by age two, photosensitivity, long limbs and large hands, mental retardation, death during second decade
Metageria	AR	Scalp hair is fine and sparse	Lack of subcutaneous fat, thin face, broad nose, mottled pigmentation and telangiectases by second decade of life
Poikiloderma Congenital (Rothmund-Thomson Syndrome)	AR	Sparse or absent scalp, axillary and pubic hair and often few eyelashes	In infancy erythema of face, ears, extensor limbs followed by mottled pigmentation, possible cataracts and hypogonadism
Progeria	AR	Normal at birth, alopecia begins at age two and progresses to total baldness	Sclerodermoid-like changes during first year, retarded somatic growth by year two, little old man and early death (arteriosclerosis)
Werner's Syndrome (Pangeria)	AR	Greying of hair at temples by age 12-14, usually complete by age 20 and followed by progressive alopecia, body hair sparse	Growth ceases by age 12, progressive sclerosis of skin over lower limbs with loss of subcutaneous fat, ulcers on legs common, generalized arteriosclerosis and high incidence of malignant disease

AR = autosomal recessive
*After Rook, A., Dawber, R.: Diseases of the Hair and Scalp (2nd ed). Oxford: Blackwell Scientific Publications, 1991:167–199.

Table 11.9 Major Congenital Hypotrichosis in Skeletal Abnormalities*

	Inheritance	Abnormal Hair	Miscellaneous
Adams-Oliver Syndrome (Aplasia Cutis with limb defects)	AD	Scalp defects at birth–solitary or multiple, heal with scarring alopecia	Incomplete formation of limbs (short toes, deficiency of phalangeal bones, syndactylism)
Cartilage Hair Hypoplasia	AR	Fine, light-colored hair, often short, silky and sparse	Dwarfism, metaphyseal dysostosis, susceptibility to infections
Chondrodysplasia Punctata (Conradi-Hunerman)	AD & XD	Coarse hair and patchy alopecia (cicatricial) hair lusterless and twisted, irregular diameter	Ichthyosis, stippled calcification of epiphyses, saddle nose, congenital cataracts, dwarfism
Focal Dermal Hypoplasia (Goltz Syndrome)	Probably XD (Lethal in male)	Sparse and brittle hair, patchy alopecia of scalp and/or pubic area	Asymmetrical linear streaks of atrophy and telangiectasia, 'fat herniations', raspberry papillomas, absent or dystrophic nails, skeletal defects, radiological findings of osteopathia striata
Hypomelia, Hypotrich-osis, Facial Hemangioma	AR	Sparse silver-blond hair	Limb reduction defects (pseudo–thalidomide syndrome), facial capillary nevus
Incontinentia Pigmenti	XD	Linear and patchy alopecia or diffuse alopecia	Defects of teeth, bones, eyes and CNS, blisters in first few months, swirls of hyperpigmentation

AD = autosomal dominant, AR = autosomal recessive, XD = sex–linked dominant
*After Rook, A., Dawber, R.: Diseases of the Hair and Scalp (2nd ed). Oxford: Blackwell Scientific Publications, 1991:167–199.

Table 11.10 Minor Hypotrichosis in Other Hereditary Syndromes*

	Inheritance	Abnormal Hair	Miscellaneous
Bazex (follicular atrophoderma and basal cell carcinomas) (unrelated to the paraneoplastic Bazex syndrome)	AD	Normal to sparse hair, hair shaft defects with pili torti	Follicular atrophoderma from birth, multiple basal cell epitheliomas from adolescence, hypohidrosis, milia
Cardio-Facio-Cutaneous Syndrome	Sporadic	Sparse, fine, brittle or thick and woolly, patchy scalp alopecia	Psychomotor and growth retardation, cardiac abnormalities, some have abnormal nails and teeth
Congenital Triangular Alopecia	Sporadic	Triangular areas of hair loss from birth in frontotemporal regions extending to frontal hairline	No associated defects known
Dyskeratosis Congentia	AD or X–linked	Often normal, may be fine dry and sparse	Normal through age five, recurrent paronychia and nail dystrophy and loss, leukoplakia, reticulate pigmentation on neck
Dystrophia Myotonica (Steinert's disease)	AD	Premature greying and frontoparietal baldness, reduction in body hair	Myotonia and muscle wasting with onset in third decade, dry skin, loss of subcutaneous fat
Encephalocraniocu–taneous Lipomatosis	Sporadic	Alopecia overlying soft scalp tumors (usually unilateral)	Lipomas of scalp, ocular lesions, unilateral cerebral malformations
Hypomelanosis of Ito (Incontinentia pigmenti achromians)		Scalp hair may be sparse	Depigmentation, ocular and dental defects
Johanson-Blizzard	Probably AR	Hypopigmented, fine, sparse hair and aplasia cutis of scalp	Multiple defects (deafness, absence of teeth, short stature, mental retardation, pancreatic insufficiency, hypothyroidism, etc.)
Pachyonychia Congenita	AD	Severe hypotrichosis in 10% of cases, kinky hair and other shaft defects	Thickening of nail bed from birth, pronounced transverse curve to nail, palmoplantar keratoderma, leukoplakia
Xeroderma Pigmentosum	AR	Usually clinically normal reported cases with absence of hair	Defect in DNA excision repair, extreme photosensitivity, pigmentation, atrophy, keratoses, malignancies

AD = autosomal dominant, AR = autosomal recessive, X-linked = sex-linked
*After Rook, A., Dawber, R.: Diseases of the Hair and Scalp (2nd ed). Oxford: Blackwell Scientific Publications, 1991:167–199.

Table 11.11 Minor Hypotrichosis in Metabolic and Other Disorders

	Inheritance	Abnormal Hair	Miscellaneous
Acrodermatitis Enteropathica	AR	Hypotrichosis to complete alopecia (banding in polarized light) rapid response to zinc	Diarrhea, acral and periorificial dermatitis, failure to thrive
Argininosuccinic Aciduria	AR	Dry with fracturing at ends, trichorrhexis nodosa, irregular growth	Mental retardation, seizures, ataxia recurrent vomiting, brittle nails
Citrullinuria	AR	Fragile with atrophic bulb, banded on microscopic exam (bamboo hair)	Mental retardation, neonatal lethargy, irritability and convulsions
Phenylketonuria	AR	Blond or light brown hair (darkens after treatment)	Normal at birth, fair skin, atopic dermatitis, untreated are mentally retarded and show abnormal neurological manifestations

AR = autosomal recessive

Table 11.12 Minor Hypotrichosis in Chromosomal Abnormalities*

	Inheritance	Abnormal Hair	Miscellaneous
Downs Trisomy 21		Normal to sparse, fine and dry, horizontal pattern of pubic hair in both sexes, alopecia areata frequent	Fixed erythema of cheeks, livedo reticularis of limbs, keratosis pilaris, unique facial appearance, mental retardation, congenital heart malformations, short limbs and fingers
Klinefelter's Syndrome	XXY	Diminished facial and body hair, sparsity of beard hair, horizontal pubic escutcheon	Delayed puberty, testes remain small, gynecomastia, some have eunuchoid body proportions

*After Rook, A., Dawber, R.: Diseases of the Hair and Scalp (2nd ed). Oxford: Blackwell Scientific Publications, 1991:167–199.

Recommended Reading

Aoyagi, T., Porter, P.S.: "Genetic disorders of hair growth: Pathogenesis of human hair defects." In: Kobori, T., Montagna, W., Toda, K., (Eds.) *Biology and Disease of the Hair.* Baltimore: University Park Press 1976;473–487.

Bergsma, D.: *Birth Defects Compendium* (2nd ed). New York: Alan R. Liss, Inc; The National Foundation–March of Dimes. 1979.

Birnbaum, P.S., Baden, H.P.: "Heritable disorders of hair." *Dermatologic Clinics,* 1987;5:137–153.

Blaustein, H.S., Stevens, A.W., Stevens, P.D.: "Rothmund-Thomson syndrome associated with annular pancreas and duodenal stenosis. A case report." *Pediatr Dermatol* 1993;10:159–163.

Boothby, C.B., Bower, B.D.: "Cartilage hair hypoplasia." *Arch Dis Childh* 1973;48:918–921.

Clarke, A., Phillips, D.I.M., Brown, R., et al.: "Clinical aspects of X-inked hypohidrotic ectodermal dysplasia." *Arch Dis Child* 1987;62:989–998.

Cunniff, C.: "Hypohidrotic ectodermal dysplasia." *Pediatr Dermatol* 1990;7:235–236.

de Luna, M.L., Raspa, M.L., Ibargoyen, J.: "Oral-facial-digital Type I syndrome of Papillon-Leage and Psaume." *Pediatr Dermatol* 1992;9:52–56.

Der Kaloustian, V.M., Kurban, A.K.: *Genetic Diseases of the Skin.* New York: Springer-Verlag; 1979.

Ellis, J., Dawber, R.P.R.: "Ectodermal dysplasia syndrome: a family study." *Clin Exp Dermatol* 1980;5:295–304.

Familusi, J.B., Jaiyesimi, F., Ojo, C.O., et al.: "Hereditary anhidrotic ectodermal dysplasia. Studies in a Nigerian family." *Arch Dis Childh* 1975;50:642–647.

Fosko, S.W., Stenn, K.S., Bolognia, J.L.: "Ectodermal dysplasias associated with clefting: Significance of scalp dermatitis." *J Am Acad Dermatol* 1992;27:249–256.

Frieden, I.J.: "Aplasia cutis congenita: a clinical review and proposal for reclassification." *J Am Acad Dermatol* 1986;14:646–660.

Freire-Maia, N., Pinheiro, M.: *Ectodermal Dysplasias: A Clinical and Genetic Study.* New York: Alan R. Liss, Inc; 1984.

Happle, R.: "Genetic defects involving the hair." In: *Hair and Hair Diseases.* Orfanos, C.E., Happle, R. (Eds). Berlin, Springer-Verlag; 1990:325–362.

Hay, R.J., Wells, R.S.: "The syndrome of ankyloblepharon, ectodermal defects and cleft lip and palate: an autosomal dominant condition." *Br J Dermatol* 1976;94:277– 289.

Halper, S., Rubenstein, D.: "Aplasia cutis congenita associated with syndactyly and supernumerary nipples: Report of a second family with similar findings." *Pediatr Dermatol* 1991;8:32–34.

Jones, K.L.: *Smith's Recognizable Patterns of Human Malformation (4th ed).* Philadelphia: W.B. Saunders Co; 1988.

Kalter, D.C., Atherton, D.J., Clayton, P.T.: "X-linked dominant Conradi-Hunerman syndrome presenting as congenital erythoderma." *J Am Acad Dermatol* 1989;21:248–256.

Ludwig, E.: "Hypotrichosis congenita hereditaria Type M. Unna." *Arch Dermatol* Syph 1953;196:261–278.

Marghoob, A.A., Orlow, S.J., Kopf, A.W.: "Syndromes associated with melanocytic nevi." *J Am Acad Dermatol* 1993;29:373–388.

McCloud, D.J., Solomon, L.M.: "The tricho-rhino-phalangeal syndrome." *Brit J Dermatol* 1977;96:403–407.

McKusick, V.A.: *Mendelian inheritance in man. Catalogs of autosomal dominant, autosomal recessive, and X-linked phenotypes.* Johns Hopkins University Press (8th ed.) Baltimore. 1988.

Micali, G., Cook, B., Blekys, I., et al.: "Structural hair abnormalities in ectodermal dysplasia." *Pediatr Dermatol* 1990;7:27–32.

Minars, N.: "Congenital temporal alopecia." *Arch Dermatol* 1974;109:395–396.

Muller, S.: "Alopecia: syndromes of genetic significance." *J Invest Dermatol* 1973;60:475–492.

O'Donnell, B.P., James, W.D.: "Rapp-Hodgkin ectodermal dysplasia." *J Am Acad Dermatol* 1992;27:323–326.

Olsen, E.A.: "Hair loss in childhood." In: *Disorders of Hair Growth. Diagnosis and Treatment,* Olsen, E.A. (Ed.). New York: McGraw-Hill 1994:139–194.

Porter, P.S., Lobitz, W.C.: "Human hair; a genetic marker." *Br J Dermatol* 1970;83:225–241.

Rajagopalan, K., Tay, C.H.: "Hidrotic ectodermal dysplasia." *Arch Dermatol* 1977;113:481–485.

Rapp, R.S., Hodgkin, W.E.: "Anhidrotic ectodermal dysplasia: autosomal dominant inheritance with palate and lip anomalies." *J Med Genet* 1968;5:269–272.

Rodini, E., Richieri-Costa, A.: "EEC syndrome: report on 20 new patients. Clinical and genetic considerations." *Am J Med Genet* 1990;37:42–53.

Rook, A., Dawber, R.: *Diseases of the Hair and Scalp (2nd ed).* Oxford: Blackwell Scientific Publications, 1991:167–199.

Solomon, L.M., Kener, E.J.: "The ectodermal dysplasias: problems of classification and some newer syndromes." *Arch Dermatol* 1980;116:1295–1299.

Toribio, J., Quinones, P.A.: "Hereditary hypotrichosis simplex of the scalp. Evidence of autosomal dominant inheritance." *Br J Dermatol* 1974;92:687–696.

Tosti, A.: "Congenital triangular alopecia. Report of fourteen cases." *J Am Acad Dermatol* 1987;16:991–993.

Traupe, H., Happle, R.: "Alopecia ichthyotica. A characteristic feature of congenital ichthyosis." *Dermatologica* 1983;167:225–230.

Vennos, E.M., Collins, M., James. W.D.: "Rothmund-Thomson syndrome: Review of the world literature." *J Am Acad Dermatol* 1992;27:750–762.

Miscellaneous Causes of Hair Loss

Definition

Alopecia may sometimes be associated with other scalp diseases or with other skin diseases involving the scalp.

Etiology

Some of the skin conditions which may be accompanied by a loss of scalp hair are listed in Table 12.1.

Clinical Features

Variable degrees of pruritus, erythema, scaling and crusting are common in these scalp disorders. Extensive alopecia is uncommon but may occur when the skin disease is severe, and particularly if it is accompanied by intense pruritus and excoriation. The alopecia is reversible following successful treatment of the underlying scalp disorder, unless permanent scarring has resulted from causes such as trauma or infection.

Seborrheic dermatitis:
Seborrheic dermatitis is a common skin disorder and can occur at any time during life from puberty onward. An infantile form of seborrheic dermatitis is seen within the first three months of life (Figure 12.1a). Seborrheic dermatitis usually presents as mild erythema and scaling which is generalized over the scalp. In more severe cases thicker, greasier crusts are seen which are usually symmetrical if not generalized. Seborrheic dermatitis may also affect eyebrows, eyelids, ears, perinasal areas and other parts of the body. The cause of seborrheic dermatitis is unknown but it may be triggered by seasonal factors, underlying bacterial or fungal infections, other debilitating illnesses, and emotional stress. The usual manifestation is persistent dandruff of varying severity, often accompanied by pruritus. There is usually no alopecia, but in severe cases, with thick crusting and excoriation, patchy or diffuse alopecia of a temporary nature may be present (Figure 12.1b).

Psoriasis:
Psoriasis is a common disease which can present at any age. In early cases the patches of erythema and scaling are generally more circumscribed than diffuse and well demarcated lesions may be seen. These lesions commonly occur on the lower occipital region of the scalp and also on the parietal areas above the ears. The clinical diagnosis of psoriasis in these lesions may be supported by the presence of a positive Auspitz sign, in that scale may be readily detachable leaving a smooth, glistening surface with pinpoint hemorrhages below. In severe cases the lesions can occur all over the scalp and may be very noticeable in the frontal and temporal areas. Sometimes a dense psoriatic crusting is present all over the scalp. Eyebrows, ears and perinasal areas may also be involved as well as the rest of the body and the nails. In many cases of psoriasis there is no alopecia, but in severe cases with crusting and adherent scales, broken

off hairs may be seen in a patchy distribution. In other cases a more diffuse hair loss is present which sometimes appears to be a telogen effluvium (Figures 12.2a,b). Note that alopecia related to psoriasis is not permanent.

Tinea (pityriasis) amiantacea:
This uncommon condition is characterized by masses of overlapping silvery scales which adhere to the scalp and are attached in layers to the hair shaft. The clinical appearance may be psoriasiform or eczematous, but the dense adherent scales are characteristic of this condition. One form is seen in young girls with current fissuring behind the ears and another form is seen in middle aged women associated with lichenified patches of scalp skin. There may be no underlying disease, but a number of cases eventually develop typical lesions of psoriasis and some take on the characteristics of a seborrheic dermatitis. The condition is chronic and hair loss is common in the areas of severe scaling (Figure 12.3). The hair regrows when the condition resolves.

Pruritus, lichenification and lichen simplex:
Pruritus of the scalp is a common complaint and is often difficult to explain. Frequently no changes are seen in the scalp skin, but causes of pruritus include seborrheic dermatitis, psoriasis, pediculosis capitis, tinea capitis, acne necrotica, other dermatoses and mental stress with anxiety and depression. An itchy scalp may be part of a generalized pruritus due to some internal cause. Simple pruritus is not usually accom-

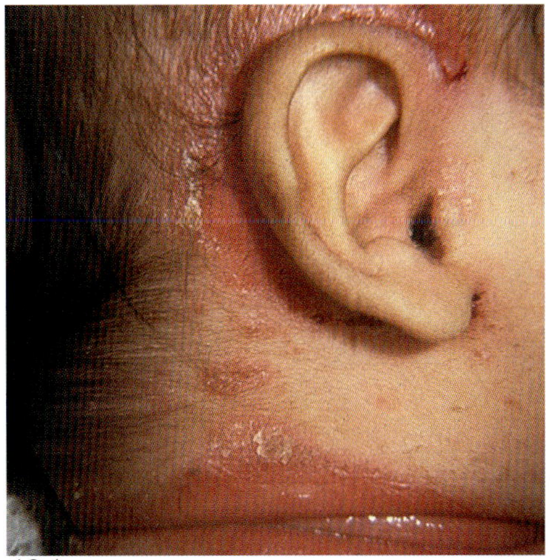
12.1a →

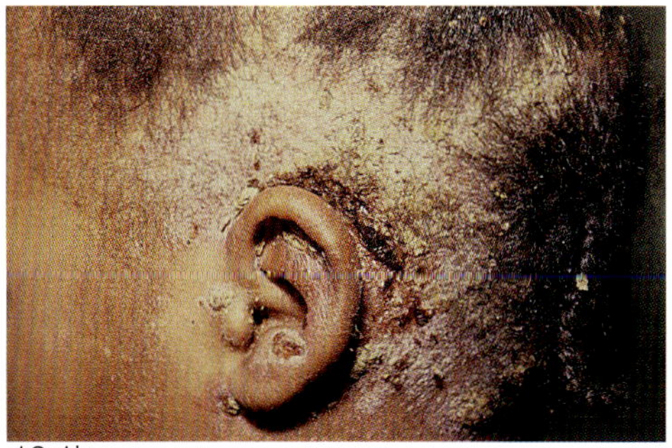
12.1b ■

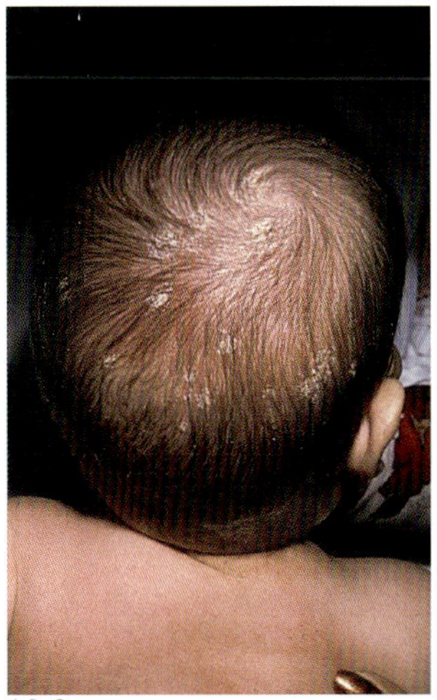
12.2a →

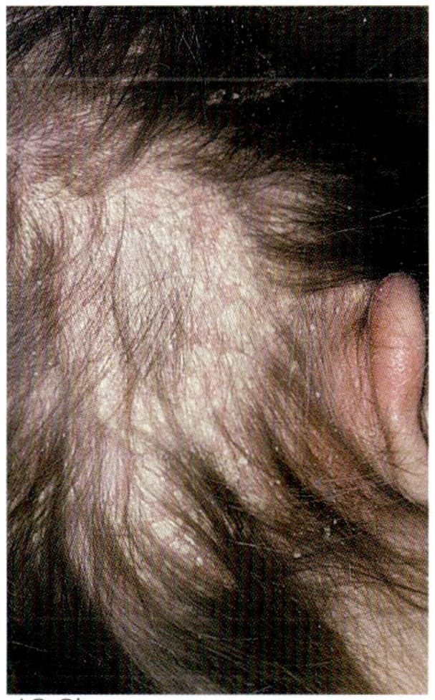
12.2b ■

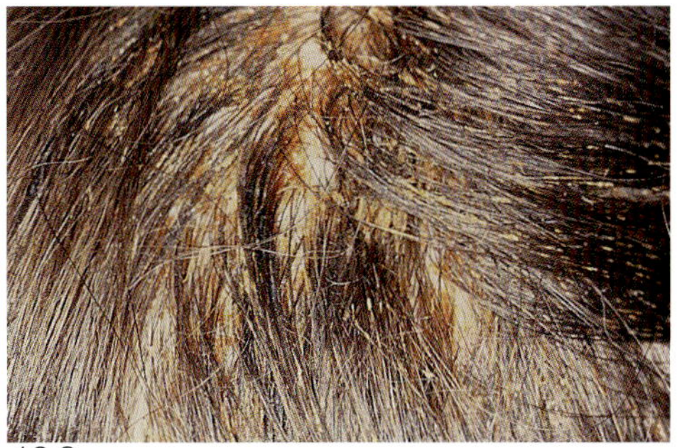
12.3

12.1
Seborrheic dermatitis:

a. Moist, eczematous lesions involve the neck folds and the perioral area, accompanied by some localized hair thinning in this infant.

b. Severe, scaly dermatitis is associated with secondary infection and patchy loss of hair.

12.2
Psoriasis:

a. Guttate psoriasis is associated with diffuse alopecia in this infant.

b. Psoriasis: Confluent psoriasis above the ear in an adult is associated with patchy hair loss.

12.3
Tinea (pityriasis) amiantacea: Dense adherent scales are associated with patchy alopecia over the posterior vertex.

panied by hair loss, but if there is prolonged scratching with lichenification (Figure 12.4a) or constant excoriation of localized areas leading to lichen simplex chronicus (Figure 12.4b), then patches of broken off hairs are common. In many cases the primary cause cannot be established and these cases are often classified as neurodermatitis.

Investigation and Diagnosis

The diagnosis can often be made on clinical grounds. A careful history is important and an examination of the skin in general and of the nails, is useful in addition to careful examination of the scalp. In some cases microscopic examination of hair and skin samples with potassium hydroxide is indicated and fungal culture may be necessary. Scalp biopsies can be useful if the diagnosis is in doubt (Figure 12.5).

Differential Diagnosis

It is important to exclude tinea capitis, pediculosis capitis, irritant or allergic contact dermatitis, simple dandruff (pityriasis capitis), acne necrotica and other forms of folliculitis, and rarer skin diseases such as dermatitis herpetiformis and Darier's disease.

Treatment

In mild cases of seborrheic dermatitis and psoriasis, simple shampoos may be adequate such as those containing selenium sulfide, zinc pyrithion, tar derivatives, and/or keratolytics such as salicylic or glycolic acid. Severe cases may require topical or intralesional steroids and any underlying bacterial or fungal infection should be treated appropriately. Grenz ray therapy is useful for pruritus of the scalp and for seborrheic dermatitis and psoriasis. ■

12.4
Excoriation:

a. Prurigo nodularis: Several prurigo papules are associated with patchy alopecia following excoriation.

b. Lichen simplex chronicus on the nape of the neck is associated with some alopecia due to broken–off hairs.

12.5
Scalp biopsy: Histopathology of seborrheic dermatitis: Vertical section: Hyperkeratosis, parakeratosis and mild spongiosis are present.

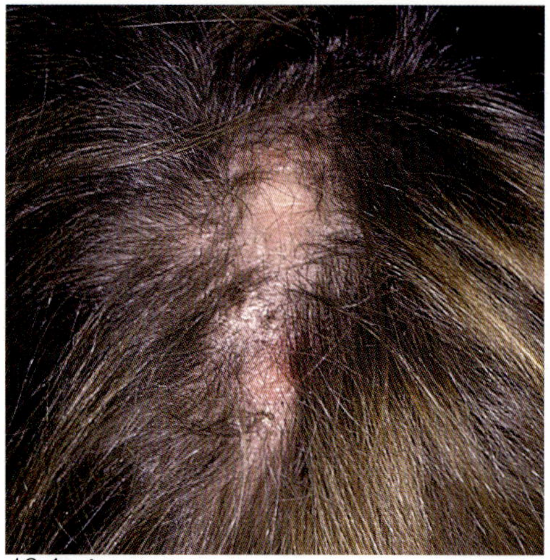

12.4a ↓

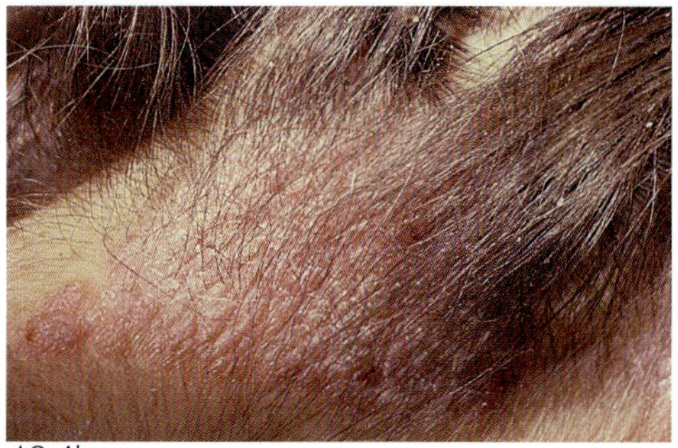

12.4b ■

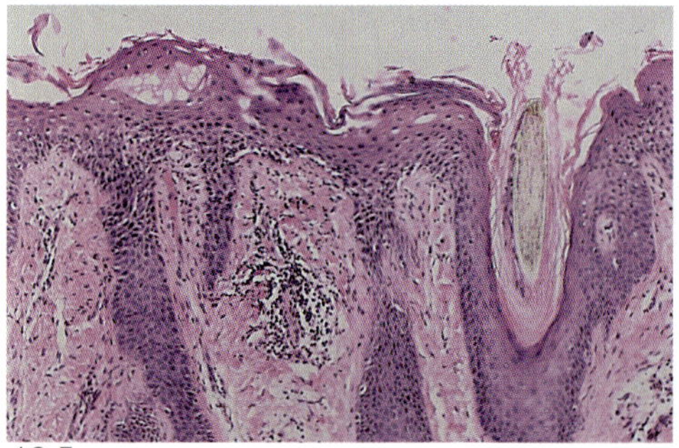

12.5

Table 12.1 Skin disorders sometimes accompanied by alopecia

Seborrheic dermatitis
Psoriasis
Tinea amiantacea
Pruritus, lichenification and lichen simplex

Suggested Reading

Brown, W.H.: "Some observations on neurodermatitis of the scalp with particular reference to tinea amiantacea." *Br J Dermatol* 1948;60:81–90.

DeVillez, R.L.: "Infections, physical, and inflammatory causes of hair and scalp abnormalities." In: *Disorders of Hair Growth. Diagnosis and Treatment,* Olsen, E.A. (Ed.). New York: McGraw-Hill 1994:83–90.

Hansted, B., Lindskov, R.: "Pityriasis amiantacea and psoriasis: a follow up study." *Dermatologica* 1983;166:314–315.

Hersle, K., Lindholm, A., Mobacker, A., et al.: "Relationship of pityriasis amiantacea to psoriasis." *Dermatologica.* 1979;159:245–250.

Keipert, J.A.: "Greasy scaling pityriasis amiantacea and alopecia: a syndrome in search of a cause." *Aust J Dermatol* 1985;26:41–44.

Knight, A.G.: "Pityriasis amiantacea: a clinical and histopathological investigation." *Clin Exp Dermatol* 1977;2:137–143.

Marks, R., Wells, G.C.: "A histochemical profile of lichen simplex." *Br J Dermatol* 1973;88:557–562.

Marks, R., Wells, G.C.:" Lichen simplex: morphodynamic correlates." *Br J Dermatol* 1973;88:249–256.

Parrish, J.A., Arndt, K.A.: "Seborrheic dermatitis of the beard." *Br J Dermatol* 1972;87:241–244.

Ring, D.S., Kaplan, D.L.: "Pityriasis aminantacea: A report of 10 cases." *Arch Dermatol* 1993;129:913–914.

Rook, A.: "Seborrheic dermatitis." *Practitioner.* 1954;172:522–530.

Rook, A., Dawber, R.: *Diseases of the Hair and Scalp* (2nd ed.), Oxford: Blackwell Scientific Publications, 1991:493–539.

Shaffer, B., Beerman, H.: "Lichen simplex chronicus and its variants." *Arch Dermatol Syphilol* 1951;64:340–351.

Shahrad, P., Marks, R.: "Hair follicle kinetics in psoriasis." *Br J Dermatol* 1976;94:7– 12.

Siemund, J.: "Alopezie bei vulgerer psoriasis der Kopfhaut. Ein Klinicher und histologischer Bericht." *Dermatol Monatsschr* 1985;171:50–57.

A

B

E

F

G

H

I

J

K

L

M

N

O

P

Q

R

S

T

U

V

W

X

Z